MW01234067

Also, By Deb Mertan

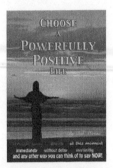

<u>A Self-Love workbook</u>
Link <u>https://www.amazon.com/-/e/B017XOLO3M</u>

Visit our website at: LoveEqualsLove.org

Loveequalslove Facebook page tiny url: **https://tinyurl.com/y82ckaa2**

Let's make a statement that "Love Equals Love" with our apparel at:
Love's Store: <u>https://www.cafepress.com/lovesstore</u>

If you enjoyed this book or found it to be life changing. I would truly appreciate it if you would post a short review on Amazon. Your support really makes a difference. I personally read all of the reviews. So I can create even better books.
Much love and appreciation,

Deb

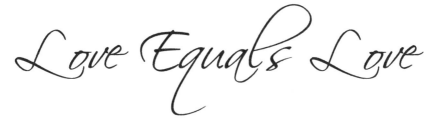

Love Equals Love

Collection of Self-Love blogs by Deb Mertan, Vol. 1

DEB MERTAN

authorHOUSE®

AuthorHouse™
1663 Liberty Drive
Bloomington, IN 47403
www.authorhouse.com
Phone: 833-262-8899

© *2020 Deb Mertan. All rights reserved.*

www.yourmemoriesrenewed.com

No part of this book may be reproduced, stored in a retrieval system, or transmitted by any means without the written permission of the author.

Published by AuthorHouse 08/07/2020

ISBN: 978-1-7283-6905-1 (sc)
ISBN: 978-1-7283-7019-4 (e)

Print information available on the last page.

Any people depicted in stock imagery provided by Getty Images are models, and such images are being used for illustrative purposes only. Certain stock imagery © Getty Images.

This book is printed on acid-free paper.

Because of the dynamic nature of the Internet, any web addresses or links contained in this book may have changed since publication and may no longer be valid. The views expressed in this work are solely those of the author and do not necessarily reflect the views of the publisher, and the publisher hereby disclaims any responsibility for them.

CONTENTS

Warning.. vii

Dedication and Appreciation...................................... ix

A Deliberate Creator 1

Attitude, Attitude, Attitude....................................... 5

Beauty is in the Eye of the Beholder 10

Don't Hang onto Residue.. 13

I Found the Fountain of Youth.................................17

Life's a Game, Aim to Win.. 21

Look for the Silver Lining 25

Looking Through Rose Colored Glasses.................... 28

Momentum... 32

One of a Kind Painting.. 36

PMS, Not What You Think 39

Re-train Your Brain... 42

Think Big, Then HUGE, Then ENORMOUS 46

Weird Like Me... 50

What Does Satisfaction Feel Like? 54

What's the Rush? 57

You're Always Here, You're Never There 60

You Be You, And I'll Be Me...................................... 63

Do Unto Others.. 66

God is Colorless 69

Shit Happens!... 73

Take What You Want and Leave the Rest 78

Tell a New Story 80

Today is Someday.. 83

Wash, Rinse, Repeat 87
What to Expect When You Love You................................. 90
You're Trying too Hard 93
Looking Through Rose Colored Glasses............................. 96
That Sneaky Doubt 100
Focus on the Good.. 104
Be Intentional 107
New Perspective.. 110
Make a Decision Already! 113
About the Author.. 117

WARNING

If you are ready to be the best you've ever been then this book is for you. But I warn you that not everything will resonate with you, so take what you want and leave the rest. But then again you might really get it and you'll love everything you read. Whatever the case, it's all good. Go forth and prosper. *I DARE YOU!*

Love,
Deb

DEDICATION AND APPRECIATION

I want to dedicate this book to all my mentors. I have never met them personally but because I have listened to them and read their works and watched their videos I feel like I do know them.

First and foremost is Abraham Hicks, infinite intelligence spoken through Ester Hicks. They are the most enlightening beings in the Universe, and I appreciate everything they have done through Ester to help us know what life is supposed to be like.

And Wayne Dyer whom I love listening to because he is such an honest and open being.

And Eckhart Tolle who teaches us how to live in the NOW.

There are many more people that talk about the Law of Attraction but these are a few of my favorites. So I want to thank them and share them with the world.

A DELIBERATE CREATOR

P lease believe me when I say that you and every single living thing on this planet are much more than this physical body that you see as you. Everything is from the source that some people might call God or your higher self or any number of beliefs that a person might have. There is definitely a spiritual side of all of us that is always with us and always wanting only wellbeing for us. If you could just wrap your head around this concept you would see just how much you have been creating by default, and how easily you could start being a deliberate creator. You can actually create the world you want to live in on purpose. When I say creating by default I mean that you are just observing what is and taking that as your reality instead of knowing that you are the boss of you and you can change your old beliefs and start believing what feels right to you and only you.

I can look back on my life now and see how things have always worked out for me. And I know that a lot of it was not conscious. But there have also been times that I was pre-paving by talking about what I wanted and not letting doubt get in the way. But even doing that was not with the knowledge of me working in concert with the Universe. I just knew I wanted whatever it was and I was sure going to find a way of letting myself have it. And what I mean by pre-paving is just keeping a positive focus on what you want, and not worrying about how long it takes to get to you in physical form. This is the working in concert part. You don't plant a seed and expect it to grow over night. You understand that there is a process and that if you tend to it properly by watering it and giving it time to grow that eventually you will have the plant that the seed turns into.

I used to live my life trying to please other people like my parents, or the teachers in school, or the government who are always trying to control

1

the masses with rules and laws that don't always have the best intentions for the masses, but are put in place to help the rich get richer and keep the rest of the people struggling. I used to think that I had no choice but to follow their rules and live a mediocre life. But now that I'm older, and I have a few experiences under my belt, I know that I can be, do or have anything and everything I want. By reading books and finding ways of uplifting my spirit from the inside out I have come to realize that the only person I need to please is me. Once I came to this conclusion I started on a journey that I know will last a life time. I know now that there is no going back. Once you get a taste of deliberate creation you can't stop. It's an addiction that you don't want to give up. I have been working on myself for years now, but it wasn't until I found out what the missing piece was to getting my life the way I wanted it to be. It is in the keeping yourself happy that makes all the difference. The way I found to stay happy a majority of the time is by not observing what was happening in the world around me and only focusing on my bliss. Oh yes, and not giving a crap about what anyone else thinks. They are not living my life. They don't know what truly makes me happy. So why are other people trying to get you to do what they think you should do? Because they are looking for love in all the wrong places. Other people think that by getting you to do what they want will show that you love them, but it usually leads to resentment, which is not a good feeling at all. Now I'm not saying you should never do things for other people, I'm saying to only do it if you really want to, otherwise say no as politely as possible.

I have a good example of someone living a life that was not in alignment with his true self. It was at a time when being gay was very taboo, and even though this person had these feelings he tried to suppress them and live a heterosexual life. After four children and ten years of marriage he finally couldn't deny it anymore. And when he did come out it turned into a nightmare. His wife was very confused and hurt and his kids didn't know what to think. His dad was so upset he wanted to kick his ass, but he never did. And because he waited so long to be true to himself he went ape shit and ended up contracting aids. I know that this story is a little extreme but it just goes to show how not allowing yourself to be true you can do more harm than good.

As it is very true that we don't all want the same things in life, which is good because that would just be nuts, it is also true that we can have, do or be anything we do want. We just have to be clear on what it is we do want and not destroy the dream with negative or contrary thoughts. And patients is a virtue. Just like the seed in the ground, once you plant it you have to know that the process is under way and all you have to do is go on with your life while it grows. Be easy about it, and don't take unnecessary action. Wait for the inspired action to come. You'll know when the time is right. There is such a thing as too much effort. Take your time and let the idea take shape before taking too much action. When you are truly following your bliss you will find that what you want comes easier and faster than you can imagine. It's almost magical. But it is the way it should be. Life is meant to be abundant in all areas. You hit the lottery in so many ways everyday of your life. Just look around at the friends you have and the love that comes from friends and family. Look around and appreciate the beauty that shows up every morning with each new sunrise. The sky is like a giant canvas and every day there is a new painting to observe and be awed by. We all have so much to be joyful about, we just have to realize it and look for the silver lining every chance we get. Life can be so delicious if we let it.

When we worry or fret we block ourselves from the good stuff that is right outside our door waiting for us to let it in. The way to let it in is to stop resisting our urges and going with the flow. The flow of life that feels good and natural. Not forced, not because we have to, but easy and joyful. Relax into life and stay calm. Give yourself permission to rest more and have fun. Speak only about what you want in your life and never look back at what was, unless you want to keep it active in your world. See only the good in other people. And if there is someone in your life that is not matching your vibe it's okay not to be around them. Your world is just that, you are the boss and no one can tell you how to live except you. Love yourself wholly. Be nice to yourself every day. And always know that the bigger part of you, your spirit, is always with you and is always willing to guide, assist, uplift and love you unconditionally. Yes, once you feel your God given power and realize that life is good there is no turning back. Being deliberate is so wonderful and awesome that once you practice yourself into your new world, you will never want to feel bad again. Yes there will be times when you may have an un-expected reaction to some situation, but it is so much easier now to pull away from those bad feelings and align with your inner being who is always seeing you as the person you are meant to be. And when I say practice I mean that this is an on-going thing that you will never get done. Because each time you reach a goal that will just cause you to set a new one. And you can't get it wrong because it is your journey to pick and choose which route you want to take. Which is again about following your bliss.

So I say to whomever is reading this blog, go forth and prosper in whatever way you choose. Be happy and always be nice to yourself. Do everything from the mindset of love and follow your intuition, or your gut as they say. If it feels good do it and be selfish enough to care about how you feel. There is much love here for you.

Sincerely,

Deb Mertan

ATTITUDE, ATTITUDE, ATTITUDE

S o everyone has ideas of what they want and why they want it. And it is my belief that we can all accomplish what most might call the impossible. And it is also my belief that it is as easy to create a castle as it is to create a button. I know that it may seem strange to a person at first, to accept these statements as truth, after all, most of us have been taught by our parent, teachers and other such authorities to think the way they do, whatever that may be. But I'm here to tell you that you have every right with full authority, by you and only you, to change the way you think, therefore changing what you choose to believe. More and more people are starting to realize that thinking positive thoughts is very beneficial, and asking for what you want is okay. And even though you may think that you have been asking for what you want to come to you, you may be sabotaging your desire inadvertently.

You may be thinking of something you want such as a new home. You are not really in a position to buy one according to what you have been observing in your life, so even though you have the desire you are also doubting that it will become a reality. You see, this causes a split in your energy and your indecision is blocking you from getting what you want. Now once you make the decision and you feel really good about it, now you're going to see forward movement. You see, it's not what you decide, it's how you feel about the decision. Is this making sense to you? Actually words don't really teach. Until you have had experiences where you have wanted something but weren't getting anxious about it, sort of like waiting for Christmas morning, there's no sense in getting all balled up wondering when it's going to get here. It's comes on the same day every year. So if we were to treat all our desires like that they could come much easier and much faster. I'm sure you could look back at a situation when something

5

like that occurred. I'll give you an example from my own life experience. My washing machine had broken down and I really didn't have an extra $500.00 to buy a new one at the moment. So I was taking my laundry to the laundromat and spending a couple of hours there every week for a couple of months. One day while hauling a ton of dirty clothes to my car, I casually said, "I have been without a washer for too long, somebodies is going to give me one." And I didn't give it another thought. My daughter happened to be with me that day, and we were having fun in an odd sort of way, but you gotta' make your own fun as far as I'm concerned. And as we were filling the 10 washers we needed, an old friend of mind called me on the phone. She asked what I was up to and I proceeded to tell her, as I was laughing about it, how we sort of took over the whole place. She said that that was why she was calling me. She had just received a large settlement from an insurance claim and she wanted to buy me a washer. I was very grateful to her, but as it was happening I knew it was me that attracted it. Things don't come out of the blue, but they can come out of the oblivious. It is so important that you care about how you feel. Think about what you're saying and how it makes you feel. Doesn't it feel yucky when you think that you are bad or not worthy? That is because that is a total untruth. We are all good and worthy. When we feel those good feelings we are on cloud 9, soaring with the eagles. When we love ourselves we can do no wrong. And no decision can be wrong when we feel good going into it. When you do decide to do something, give it your full attention. But let it gestate and grow fully in your mind and wait for the feeling of the inspired idea before you take action.

This is about attitude. No, it's about total attitude! When you have the attitude of joy and happiness things like that just keep showing up in your life. You know I gave you the example of the washing machine manifesting in a matter of minutes, but I also manifested buying a house the same way. It all started when my landlady called and said she wanted to sell the house I had been renting from her for the last three years at that point. I told her that it was cool and that I would start looking for a new place to rent. She kept apologizing but I wasn't worried about anything. I just kept the attitude that everything is always working out for me, and I kept appreciating that we had been here for this time and how much I liked this house and that I was sure we would find something just like it, or better. But things were not turning out the way I thought they would, but still I knew something good was going to happen. As people were coming through the house I was living in for the showing I was telling all the potential buyers how lovely the neighborhood was and how great the front porch is for sitting and drinking coffee in the mornings. Finally they had a buyer and I still had not found a place to rent. But I was not worried. My family was a little worried but I just kept saying that everything is going to work out just right. One day while driving I saw a sign that said $1500.00 will get you into your own home. I took the number down and gave them a call. I got an appointment right away and found out that by myself I could only qualify for a loan of $120,000.00. Well that was not going to get me the home I wanted and deserved. So they asked me if one of my kids could buy it with me. I told them that my daughter had just started a new job so she didn't qualify and my son just started a new job after going to college for 4 years. They said that if he is a graduate and if he has his diploma and transcripts and a letter from his new outstanding job that he could qualify for $250,000.00. So now we were seriously looking for a house buy, but as it turned out, together my son and I made a $1,000.00 too much to qualify for the $1,500.00 down payment program and now they wanted about $20,000.00 down and we didn't have it. Believe it or not I did not wavier from my thought that we were going to buy a house that we really loved. So the man that was buying the house that I was living in came with the inspector to do the final inspection while they were waiting for escrow to close. I was very nice to them as they crawled up into the attic and looked in all my cupboards and checked every nook and cranny they could find. After they left I called the landlady to let her know they had done their job. And for some reason I said to her, "You know, my son and I are looking to buy a house now. Too bad we can't buy this one." I told her about the down payment issue we were having too. But not because I thought she could do anything about that. I really don't know why I said it. But she said that they had signed a contract with the other people and that they would have to cancel on her. But I still didn't stop my good feeling that something magnificent was happening.

Now here's where it really starts getting good. That very night my landlady called and said that the couple that wanted the house had backed out. Again I was grateful but I knew that it was happening just the way it was supposed to happen. She also told me that she had talked to her realtor who had a very good loan officer she worked with and they said that if they raised the price of the house a little I could use that as part of the down payment. I would still need to come up with $10,000.00 but that was okay. I knew if I could manifest all that I had so far, that I could manifest the rest. So I asked for a 60 day escrow so that I could come up with the money. This just happened to be during the holiday season. We were scheduled to close escrow on December 27TH. Here it was Thanksgiving weekend and I still had not one dime toward the $10,000.00. My son was a little concerned because he didn't understand how I was so calm about everything. I just kept reassuring him that everything was going in the right direction. The whole Thanksgiving weekend I thought about who I could ask to loan me the money and one person kept popping up in my mind. So on Monday morning I gave this person a call and explained the situation to him and without one iota of hesitation he said, I think that will work. And not only did he say yes he also said it was a gift. As I hung up the phone I broke out into the most joyous tears of relief. It was so delicious to hear those words come out of his mouth. So because I stayed true to my desire and did not put any doubt on my path I was a homeowner within 2 months.

So, what are we talking about here? We're talking about staying in the attitude of joy and knowing that everything is always working out. That it is our right to be deserving and worthy. And we are the only ones that need to make ourselves happy. It is not anyone else's job to make you happy. We are all responsible for our own feelings whether they are good or bad. So if I were you I would choose to feel good. Everything is a choice so make it and live it. And know that you are the creator of you and you can re-invent you anytime you choose to. Life is meant to be good and fun and joyous. You get one shot at this one so make it a good one. Be nicer to yourself and then watch how the right people start showing up around you that will enhance your happiness. It all starts on the inside. Love comes from within and then pours out onto the world and brings it back in miraculous ways. But that's how life is supposed to be. So now that you know it, live it. You will find out that fun is the name of the game and winning is a givin'. Go forth from this day on and love yourself like you never did before. You're going to dig it. And remember there is great love here for you as well.

Until next time, your friend,

Deb Mertan

BEAUTY IS IN THE EYE OF THE BEHOLDER

Beauty is in the eye of the beholder, and the main beholder is you. When you feel beautiful, you will look beautiful. It's like having the ugliest little Chihuahua, she's blind, has hardly any teeth and sheds like a beast. You think to yourself, "How could I ever love this thing?" But as time goes on you start to notice all the little things she does that make you laugh, and how she cuddles with you when you're watching T.V. together. Before you know it you are in love and she's the most beautiful dog in the world. That is how we are supposed to look at ourselves. We need to find the good stuff, like how funny we are, if applicable, or how sweet we are. We need to be the people we want to be and that alone will help us like ourselves more. We need to treat ourselves with kindness and not freak out when we make mistakes. Mistakes could turn out to be good, look at Plexiglass or penicillin, they were accidents but they turned out to be great! Not everyone is born looking like the Princess Grace of Monaco, she was a true beauty, inside and out. And of course there are those really beautiful people that don't even know that they are because someone has convinced them otherwise. For those of us that are more regular, there are many ways to show the true beauty that is in all of us.

Now in order to find your true beauty there are a few simple steps you could take to start the process. It involves looking inward and looking for all the things you love about yourself. This is a form of self-love that will definitely stir up more thoughts and feelings about the things you love about you. And even if a person is beautiful on the outside but has a bad attitude they seem ugly to other people. Not everyone sees the same thing when they look at the same person either. For example I think the actress, Kim Basinger is beautiful, but my brother says no she's not. Of course we don't know her personally but from what we can see we both have different perspectives. But my brother also thinks the actress Daryl Hannah is gorgeous and I really don't. So you see it is all personal preference. I'm sure if we got to know those two ladies we would both change our views according to how they acted in real life. Personalities are very important in the way people view others. You can meet someone and at first glance think that they are hideous but after even a few minutes you can change your point of view just by talking to them and seeing that they are a truly kind and beautiful person. It happens!

You're probably wondering why I even brought this up. But the truth of the matter is I have not always felt so beautiful. Not that I thought I was horribly ugly, but I didn't think I was any more than average. After starting a regimen of self-love I started seeing myself in a whole new light. I started taking more pride in the way I dressed and the way I talked about myself. I stopped saying anything negative, such as I'm so stupid or I'm fat or anything that would bring my spirits down. When I would catch myself saying things like that I would immediately change it to something positive, like, I'm not stupid, just ignorant of the facts. Or, I'm not fat, I'm a beautiful woman on my way to becoming an even more beautiful woman. Of course at first this sounds foreign to someone that is not used to saying nice things to their self, but in time as you keep changing the negative to a positive whenever you catch yourself, it becomes easier and more comfortable. Practice, practice, practice. That is the remedy for anything you want to change in your life. Little by little if you start and keep using these techniques you will notice how by you caring more about you other people will too. Not only adults but even the smallest of babies will notice your beauty and want to make eye contact with you. You may even draw a big smile from them. Not to mention the animals that will see you as a very fascinating person and want to warm up to you. You see, it all starts with you. How do you want to be treated? Treat yourself the way you want to be treated and everyone else will treat you that way too.

When you are busy being nice to yourself it doesn't leave much time for finding fault with anyone else so your relationships with your loved ones will automatically improve as well. You may even become an example to others on how to become happier in their own existence. It really becomes great fun when you stop beating yourself up about things you can't change or have any control over. Look for ways to see the real you and ignore the things that make you feel bad. Life is wonderful when you look for the fun and live as happily as you can every day.

So if you are ready, show the world your beauty by starting with showing yourself your true beauty. It is not hard to do, you just have to want to do it. Be brave and look into your soul and bring out the true you so that everyone can see what a terrific person you are. Love yourself like a fat kid loves cake and life will just keep getting better and better. And never forget that there is great love here for you. So until we meet again.

With all my love,

Deb Mertan

DON'T HANG ONTO RESIDUE

My life has been pretty good lately. I have really resonated with the fact that this is an attraction based Universe. I have proven it to myself over and over again in the past couple of years. So when I started noticing money missing from my bank account it really freaked me out. How could this be happening? I have been working on my happiness and getting a lot of good results. Things seemed to be moving in a very positive direction, so why now was this happening? Well after 4 weeks of this I finally broke down and changed my account number and did all the necessary things to get everything back on track, like getting my direct deposits transferred and my automatic bill paying going again. It was a little bit of a hassle but it was worth it. I also got on line banking started which I thought I never would. During all the turmoil I couldn't get a grasp on why this was happening but now that it was taken care of I looked back at what I may have done to bring this on to myself. I had to be thinking of something that would be making this come to me. Like I said this is an attraction based Universe so whatever you focus on, good or bad, will come to you. Then I realized that while I was daydreaming about the day my millions of dollars would arrive, not how or when or who would bring it, just fantasizing about what I would buy and the trips I would take and so on, but in the back of my mind there was this soft whisper saying, but how do I keep track of all that money? It wasn't a deep thought, it was casual, just a sparse passing thought. But those are the ones that sneak up on you. It could be a good passing thought or a bad passing thought, but none the less it is sneaky.

For example, one day I was cleaning out my garage. I had loaned out one of my favorite CD's to a friend and I thought to myself that I should buy a second one so that while that one was out I could still have one to

13

listen to. As soon as the thought left my mind I opened a bag and viola there was a brand new set of the exact one I had loaned out. It was my son's but he didn't have a CD player so he left it in a bag that somehow ended up in the garage.

Now that may seem like a coincidence but these things just keep happening. Another time I had just gotten my washing machine fixed and I made the statement that the next thing I was going to get was a refrigerator. Mine was not staying cold and the freezer was thawing and re-freezing everything so that it was all frost bitten. And again I didn't say how I was going to get one or if it would be new or used, I just casually said in a matter of fact attitude that my next thing would be a refrigerator. Two days later my roommate said that his parents had sold their rental home that was very close to me and there was a refrigerator there if we wanted it. He asked me if I did want it and without hesitation I said yes, anything was better than mine. So I went to work not really thinking about what it would be like, in fact I even forgot that it was coming. When I got home I went to the coffee machine to get a cup and when I turned to get the creamer I was surprised and delighted to see a side-by-side huge white refrigerator standing there. What was really funny is that it was exactly the kind of frig that I had been wanting. And it was nice and cold inside. I literally screamed and jumped for joy.

So getting back to my story about the bank, I thought that after figuring out what had caused this, my casual thought about managing money that everything was fine and dandy once again. But gradually I started feeling pain in my right shoulder. It wasn't too bad at first but it just kept nagging at me. It was hard to sleep and it eventually started affecting my left shoulder. I was going for massages trying to sooth it and my therapist said it was affecting my whole shoulder girdle. I tried topical pain creams and ibuprofen, sitting in the spa but nothing seemed to help. So one day while listening to one of my CD's on Law of Attraction there was a story of a woman with pain from arthritis in her hips. She couldn't understand how she could think positive thoughts when she hurt so badly. It was suggested to her that she could be in pain and feel fearful or be hopeful. It is all about vibration. She was asked, how does it make you feel? The woman answered that she felt restricted and weak. Right then I realized that I was feeling that too. This whole business of being violated made me feel that way and even though it was taken care of I had not let go completely of the fear. It was residual residue that I had been hanging on to. Now you may not believe this but as soon as I realized what was going on the pain almost completely disappeared. I was astonished. It was literally instantaneous. It has been three days now and I have not used any pain relievers, no heating pad or any other type of relief and I feel great. I can sleep and work and even though I still feel a tinge of the pain that was there occasionally it is nothing I can't handle. Each passing day gets better and I have no doubt that it will continue to do so. The pain was just residual pain that I had not eliminated yet.

That actually reminded me of my mother and how she would be so calm in a crisis, but after everything would subside she would break down and cry. Now I know how that can build up and if you don't relieve it, it will show up in other ways like pain. So next time you have a back ache or any other kind of pain think about what you have been thinking about and see how fast you feel better. Then you will also know not to think that thought any more. I know this sounds simple, but that is it. The work is to think better thoughts until they become habit or new beliefs. Do this until you get so good at it that bad thoughts will just feel wrong and you will want to go back to good thoughts. You will become addicted to feeling good and you will never be able to go the other way for very long again. The momentum of the joy you create for yourself will surely turn your life around and things will just keep getting better.

As I am seeing, by life experiences, that we definitely do live in an attraction based Universe, my choices keep getting more and more deliberate. As per request so to speak. Science has proven that humans use a very small portion of their brains or minds if you will. I think the key is to make your request to the Universe or whomever you consider to be the source from which all good comes, then sit back and relax and let the Universe do its thing to bring it to you. When you finally realize that life is supposed to be easy, you will feel like a magician, conjuring up a world that pleases you immensely and exclusively. You know it's not the destination that is so delicious, it's the journey. If you really pay attention to the signs that are being revealed to you constantly, you will start to have wonderful adventures all along your path. And if you really think about it, once you do accomplish whatever it is you are after, it becomes old news and a new idea catches your eye and there you go off to the next adventure. Life is so fun when you let it be. You are the only one blocking anything from coming to you, whether it is a lover or a big pile of money or anything else you are wanting. Relax, stop trying so hard to make things happen. Realize that once you ask for something you want there is a buffer of time before it will materialize. You don't plant a seed and expect it to grow right away. So let the Universe do its job and just enjoy the process. And notice the unfolding as you move into the direction of what you want. It's not about being patient either. It's about giving it time to grow. You don't get pregnant and expect the baby to come now. You know it has to develop over a nine month period. So let your desires grow too. And have fun while waiting for the delivery. And stop doubting too. When you ask for something then question how it's going to come and when it's going to come and who is going to bring it, you add resistance to your desire and that slows everything way down and sometimes even stops the flow. So just ask and trust and go do something fun while you are waiting for whatever it is you are wanting. Expect it will come just like you know Christmas will come.

Here, let me show you an example of how to really get started. Think of yourself at the ocean. You want to go in the water but it's very cold, so you tippy toe in maybe up to your ankles, but then you back up a little so it's not so cold. Then you go back in and this time you go a little further, maybe to your shins, but it's still too cold. You keep this up until you are fully in the water and you have acclimated to the temperature. That's how learning how to change old habits or beliefs is. You do it a little at a time until it becomes normal to you. That's how you stop doubting and start believing and eventually start knowing. Life will teach you through experience so pay attention to how you speak, think and feel. You will be amazed at how wonderful and delicious your life can and will be. Go big and do great things. That's an order, so go. And remember there is great love here for you.

Forever your friend,
Deb Mertan

I FOUND THE FOUNTAIN OF YOUTH

I guess it may sound like a fairy tale to most people, that there could be a fountain of youth. But that is because they, whomever they are, have been looking for it in the outer world, when in reality it has been on the inside this entire time. Yes since the beginning of time we have had access to it and I just now figured it out for myself. Actually I have always been in touch with my inner child. I would be the adult that would be outside playing hop scotch and kick ball with all my nieces and nephews. At the time I really didn't give it much thought, I was just having fun. Oh yes, other adults thought I was silly, but who cares what they think, right? I also really love dancing. I'll be the first one on the dance floor even if I don't have a partner. I just go off into my own little world and do what I love. And I sing loudly even if it doesn't sound good to others, because it's joyous to me. Haven't you ever watched a little kid when they're at the grocery store with their mom? They just sing and dance and enjoy their selves. They aren't worried about who's watching, they're just having fun. They have the key. I guess what I am trying to get across to you is that even though we age on the outside and we will for sure die someday, which I believe is a myth because we are all energy and we just transition to another dimension, we still have the choice to be young on the inside. I still feel like I'm in my twenties and I am way past that humanly. I think I just made that word up, but I like it so it stays. I see people that are humanly younger than me but have maybe half the energy and spunk that I do. Yes for a while there I fell into the belief that you should act your age, but after my husband transitioned and I found myself single again I decided to do all the things I have been wanting to do and just never did.

So now I'm doing all sorts of fun things, like stand-up comedy for instance. I really don't care if I make a career out of it, I do it for the fun. And I also go to clubs where I dance and play and make lots of new friends. Oh, I tried karaoke once but it wasn't my thing. But at least I tried. I may do it again someday but it really doesn't matter. Life is too short to take anything too seriously. You've heard the saying, "Don't sweat the small stuff, and it's all small stuff." If you really, really, really think about it, that is the truest statement you can ever hear. What does worry accomplish anyway? It gives you wrinkles and gray hair. It causes ulcers and other illnesses, and shortens lives because stress is the silent killer. So just knowing that, doesn't it make you want you kick your shoes off and yell, I'm free, I'm free and I'll never be caged again? Well once you get past the point of guilt for not conforming to anyone else's rules, and the worry and stress that has been bogging you down, you will feel free. And that's when the inner child inside you will lead you to do anything and everything you want to do. Did you get that? I said everything you WANT to do. Want, want, want! Stop *having* to do anything. Stop using the word have. Sure there are things we do out of responsibility like paying the bills and feeding the kids, but those things can be done joyously too. Slow down and give yourself permission to be happy.

Have you ever heard the saying "The hurrier I go, the behinder I get"? Well, it is a saying and it is true. When you are rushing around and getting all twirled up in day to day tasks, you end up getting nowhere. But when you do things with an attitude of ease things flow and you can accomplish more than you thought you could. But, so what if you don't accomplish anything? You've got to stop punishing yourself for leaving dishes in the sink or because you didn't make your bed. Those things will still be there when you are ready to do them. Stop being so ridged and flow more often. Stop being so profoundly human, which to me means stiff and boring. Be more spiritual, which to me means free and fun. Life is supposed to be joyous so say yes more often. Yes I will go to the movies on a weeknight, yes I will take a weekend cruise, and yes I will act silly even if others around me scoff. Be who you *WANT* to be. There is no judge in the sky tallying up all your Brownie points. You will not make marks on some sort of chart that will get you a good seat in heaven. Now is what counts. Wouldn't it be a shame if you got really old and then looked back and asked yourself, "Why didn't I do that or I should have done this"? Yes, it would be.

Now I ask you, what is wrong with being nice to yourself? You want others to be nice to you, right? You need to sooth yourself into happiness. Take the time to get your nails done "guilt free", or take a bubble bath in the middle of the day "just because". Heck, take a nap if it feels good. Treat yourself like your own best friend. Love yourself like you do your lover. You do deserve these things and you need to see yourself as the worthy being that you truly are. You are not just a human being but a spiritual being as well. When you finally decide, and yes it is a choice, to be nice to yourself, then everything else will just fall into place. I mean everything, money, lovers, and that great vacation you've always wanted to take. All these things are available to us all the time but we get too bound up in "Reality" to see it. Stop being so reality oriented and dream more often. Believe that anything is possible and it will be for you. Slow down and meditate more, or pet your cat more often, or take a walk in a beautiful garden. See through your spiritual eyes and know that all is well. I know that deep down you know that you are always taken care of. I know you can think back to a time when you needed money for something and when you finally gave up looking for it because that was the only thing left to do, the money miraculously came. Tell me you never felt that. Well that is how it is all the time when you finally give up the struggle and let life live you. Follow the prompts like you would on a video game. Look for the signs that are always being revealed to you, be aware, be awake to the life you want and deserve. Be so in love with yourself that none of the outside bullshit can get to you. It will just roll off your back or go around you like you have a protective shield over you. Life is supposed to be fun and it would be a shame if you let it get away. Be happy in your NOW, because now is all we have. Wherever you are is okay. It's just the launching point to the next now and the next one. And when you don't get carried away with the what-ifs you will be much happier.

So how do you get to the fountain of youth? You slow down, you take it easy, and relax more, and pet your cat more, and take more walks and take more naps. Be nicer to yourself and love yourself and everything and everyone unconditionally. Be satisfied with where you are now and be eager for more. Let your inner child out more often.

So now you know the secret to the fountain of youth. It's there if you

Deb Mertan

choose to see and apply it. The ball is in your court. So what are you going to do NOW?

Remember there is great love here for you.

Always, your friend,
Deb Mertan

20

LIFE'S A GAME, AIM TO WIN

'm pretty sure that if you are on this planet you have seen, or at least heard of the movie, "Mary Poppins". One of my most favorite scenes in that movie is when Mary takes the children into the nursery and shows them how to have fun while cleaning it up. Of course in the movie all they have to do is snap their fingers and all the toys, clothes and beds covers go back to their proper places and then it's off to the park for an afternoon of chalk painting adventures. Really if you haven't seen "Mary Poppins" you should. It is truly a fantastic movie. Yes this is all fantasy but behind all the seemingly magic things that Mary Poppins can do there is a very important message. Life is supposed to be fun. And when you really look for it you will find it.

When I say life is a game, aim to win, I don't mean like a race or a competition, I mean you will win every time if you let yourself have fun and stop taking life so seriously. You know being too serious could cause stress which in turn could cause illness or disease, or even a shortening of one's life. And as far as I can tell stress is a useless emotion, except for the fact that it is a warning sign that fun is nowhere in sight. It doesn't really accomplish anything. It actually makes things worse. But there are ways to relieve stress and one way is to try to find the fun in everything you do. When you practice this you will see how useless stress is and you will never want to entertain that emotion again. Yes it takes practice, but so does everything, even being stressed all the time is a practice. You just need to be more conscious of where your emotions or thoughts are taking you. You need to take the reigns and guide yourself into the emotions that feel good to you. Be totally awake and aware of where you are headed. It's like you wouldn't get in your car and put on a blind fold and then start the engine, put it in drive and then gun it so that you take off like a rocket.

That would be ludicrous. But when you are not paying attention to your feelings and emotions that is exactly what you are doing. You would be banging into trees and other cars on the road and maybe even veering off into a ditch, and then blaming it on someone or something else. But once you take the blind fold off you can go as fast as you want to because you can maneuver around the trees and cars and avoid the ditches. Yes it is that easy to take control of your own life. Just take the blinders off and pay attention to how you feel about everything.

Now that I have figured this out my life has become so enjoyable that nothing seems to bother me anymore. I look at every so called problem with new eyes, so to speak. I start thinking about solutions immediately instead of dwelling on the situation. I love more, care more and laugh more. And when someone tells me, "Have fun tonight", as I'm going out the door, I say, "I always do". It's true, I always have a good time because the only expectation I have is to have fun.

So now that I have been paying attention to my emotions on a full time basis I can see that all I have to do is be mindful of how I feel. And yes to me it is a game and I do aim to win. I aim to win by always having a smile on my face, and seeing the joy in people's eyes when we meet and getting my face licked by my friends dogs, especially the ones that don't usually care for other people. This is proof to me that by being happy and playful the dogs can feel it too, it's feedback to let me know that I am on a good path. It really makes me feel special. I know that it might seem silly to you but I have never really been into dogs and cats as far as having one for a pet. But after keeping myself in this high flying vibration, animals have really started to gravitate to me and me to them. Even the owners are baffled by their animal's behavior toward me, but I know why it is so. That's part of the game too. I don't need to explain to anyone why their animals love me, it's our little secret, and I love it. But if someone were to ask me why I am so happy all the time I would tell them this, "I am happy because I choose to be", I make the choice every day to look for the fun in life. I look for the beauty in the trees and the flowers and in the faces of little children that still seem to know that life is supposed to be fun." You know it wouldn't be a bad idea if you were to think more like a child. Remember how fun it used to be to swing on a swing set or the monkey bars at the park or to play hide and seek with your friends, and not feel stressed out about anything, because you always knew you were safe? Maybe some people didn't feel that way but that too is the beauty of making the decision to be happy now. You see you and only you have the right to feel whatever you choose to feel. You are the boss of you and you are worthy beings. So if you are ready to start living the life you deserve then why not start having fun now? You can make anything a game. Even driving in traffic can be fun if you find a way of enjoying yourself. No one else even has to know you are playing a game. I like to count all the "Swift" trucks I can find on the road. And try saying swift without smiling. Or I like to try and see how many words I can make out of the letters on the license plates on the other cars around me. Like Mary Poppins says, when you find the element of fun the chore is a snap, or something like that, you get the gist. Or when you are cleaning your house and you always do the same routine, switch it up and see if you get finished faster by starting in a different place then you usually do. Be creative and get those juices flowing. When you have your mind on looking for the fun you won't have time to be worried or stressed out about anything, at least for the time you are playing.

Life IS supposed to be fun and we have all taken it too seriously. Just think of all we've missed out on while trying to be so serious and adult like. But don't think too long on that, just realize that it's never too late to change the game. Why not just stay a kid in a grown up body?

I'm not saying to ignore responsibility, I'm saying be responsible and have fun doing it. Sing while you're doing the dishes and dance while you're mopping the floor. Have you ever seen the movie, "Honey I Shrunk the Kids"? The daughter is dancing as she's mopping the kitchen floor and the neighbor boy is watching her through the window. He doesn't see her as dumb or stupid, he is enjoying the view. That is how people will see you once you start having fun. And even if there is someone who scoffs at you for being excessively happy, it's only because they themselves are extremely unhappy and can't understand what you are doing. I would just ignore them because they will either get on board with you or go away from you, so there is no need to worry. You are you, a unique individual, and you are the only person you need to take care of. And once you get that life will be so delicious that no one else will be able to buck your current of joy.

Now you know what's what. And you can start finding ways of playing games that you not only win, but that give you a way to share your joy with others. And you will be teaching through your examples that life is good and you can have it all. No matter where you are starting from emotionally you can always find a way to feel a little better and then a little more and before you know it you're almost always happy. And on the rare occasions that you find yourself dipping down you will know what to do about it. Sometimes it's just best to crash and burn and let the feeling pass through you. Then as you go to bed remind yourself that tomorrow is another day and you can press the reset button upon awaking the next morning. Lay there for a few minutes and think about what fun you will have that day. Pre-set your mood for the day so that if there is anything negative out there you won't even notice it. Or if you do happen to notice it, it won't bother you like it once did. You may even become the solution person because you are so in tune with life that you instinctively know how to handle just about anything with grace and ease. Maybe the next time you see your kids, or your friend's kids if you don't have any, playing in the yard you should join them, and bring back some of the memories of playful freedom. I love taking my 3 year old great niece to the store because while we're shopping she wants to skip down the aisles. So we hold hands and skip and sing. People always smile at us so I know they feel the joy we are feeling, at least in that moment.

Okay so now you know that having fun and playing games are very important for your well-being, don't you? So what's stopping you? Go out there and look for every fun thing there is to do. And believe me when you purposely look for it you will find it. And you are going to be amazed at how wonderful you feel all day every day when fun is your main goal. And do you want to know a secret about having fun? It will bring you new ideas and inspirations to be do or have anything you want in life. When you take care of you and stop worrying about ANYONE else, as far as opinions go, you will be floating on air, living *La Vida Loca*, which is Spanish for the crazy life. People are going to want to know your secret and you can say, life is a game and I aim to win. Then smile and skip away.

Remember there is always great love here for you.

Your friend,
Deb Mertan

24

LOOK FOR THE SILVER LINING

Have you ever had things going terribly wrong only to find out later that whatever it was that happened turned out to be a blessing in disguise? That is because we are always receiving what we focus on the most. Whether we want it or not, if we give it our full attention it will surely show up. You see, we live in an attraction based Universe, so when you say yes about something, and you let it gestate long enough, without adding any doubt into the mix, you will see it. But if you say no to something you don't want, you will also attract that, because you give your attention to it. The Universe doesn't hear what you say, it responds to how you feel. Example, when a parent is yelling at a child, saying in a loud voice, *"Don't you know I love you!"* it sends a mixed message to the child. The words don't match the feeling behind them. Or if you were to tell someone that you are sorry for something you did or didn't do, and you sounded snotty while saying it, that would also not match. Those are two examples of feeling verses words but it also applies to how you feel when you say you want something. Like let's say you wanted a new car and you casually said, "I'm thinking about getting a new car." You don't really hear any resistance in that statement. You could just go about your business and not give it too much thought and before you know it you would be getting a new car. But if you were to say after that statement, "But I don't see how I could do that" that would throw up a wall that would stop all momentum from moving forward. When you feel light and confident about it things move along at just the right pace. Things come to you when you are ready to receive them. But when you are all balled up asking, where is it, when is it going to get here, you slow everything way down.

Have you ever heard the phrase, ask and it is given? Well that is the truest statement ever uttered out of anyone's mouth. Sometimes you may think that what you asked for isn't coming, so you keep asking for the same thing over and over again. Being redundant doesn't help anything. The Universe knows what you want and knows how to get it to you. Just relax and be casual about it. Life is supposed to be fun and if you remember that every day you will start to see a tipping of the scale, from the not wanted to the wanted. But in order to stop thinking about the unwanted you have to start thinking about something else. You can't just stop thinking about that thing you're not going to think about. That just keeps perpetuating the thought. You have to look for things to think about or focus on that are pleasing to you, things that make you smile. Of course this all takes practice. Everything that is worth doing does take practice. Everything that you do now took training, and I mean everything, from dressing yourself to driving a car. So why is this any different? A belief is just a thought you keep thinking so why not change the direction of your thoughts. The only reason it may seem difficult at first to think better thoughts is because you have been trained either by others or by your own habits of thoughts to think that way and you have a momentum going in that direction. But if you think of your emotions or in other words your feelings, as your navigational guide you will always know which way you are going. It's like your GPS system guiding you turn by turn and when you stray it says, "Please return to the highlighted route." That is what gut instinct is all about. When you practice this and get pretty good at it you will become super sensitive to how you are feeling and be able to return to the route very quickly, before you get any momentum going in the wrong direction. This is all very simple stuff but it can seem hard at first like I mentioned earlier. And just because it seems too simple to have any effect on your mood or attitude, don't be fooled. It will have a great impact on your life in a very positive way. It can be as soon as tomorrow or it could take 30 days, it's all up to you and how earnest you are in focusing on what it is you want in your life.

Have you ever seen a 3-D printer at work? They are so awesome, and a little weird if you ask me. I have a friend that has one and I watched it make a cover for a remote control device that goes to his drone camera. As I was seeing this thing form right before my very eyes I started thinking about things working out for me in a similar way. It's like I put my request out to the Universe and then I just kick back and let it do it's thing. I don't have to keep checking to see if it's on track because I know it will work on it until all of a sudden there it is. Actually it's also like planting a seed. You don't plant corn and then get a rose bush. You know that when you plant the corn seed you will eventually get corn, but only after it takes root and grows into a full blown corn stalk. My suggestion is to know what you want and tell the story the way you want it to be. I know Donald Trump is an odd duck but he has the right idea about how to go about getting what he wants. When he is building a new building, like a casino, he talks about how great it's going to be and how everyone is going to love going there, and so on. He tells the story he wants to be true. You know you can do that with everything in your life, even the stuff you consider really bad. If you just look at things from your past with a new perspective and find the silver lining, you will feel a whole lot better and things in your now will be able to move forward. And if you don't get yourself to far into the future with what-if thoughts you will also feel a whole lot better and things will move even faster to get you to where you what to be, or should I say where you want to feel, and that just comes down to staying in a good mood and mostly being happy. You can choose to be happy right now if you really want to. You are so free to choose what you want you could choose bondage. But why would you choose something that goes against your nature to feel good? I'll tell you why, because you just got used to it, but now it's time for a change! It's time to think on purpose and create your own journey, the way you want it to be. Be your own boss and love with all your heart. Be un-conditional and love even the haters. You don't have to like or dislike anything anyone else does or doesn't do but love is a powerful tool that can spread to even the worst people on earth. If more people did more things out of love the world would have to change to a greater place to live. We all have a say in our own lives and our own world.

I guess I've rambled on long enough. If you're going to get it I'm sure you have by now. Just one last thing before I go, be careful what you wish for because you will get it, whether it's wanted or un-wanted. Be nice to yourself and love deeply. Sooner than you think things are going to change and the better it gets, the better it gets. There is great love here for you.

Forever, Your Friend
Deb Mertan

LOOKING THROUGH ROSE COLORED GLASSES

I know most people think that they need to look at what is and react to it whether it is something wanted or something unwanted. But the truth is that we all have a choice to react in any manner we desire. We honestly do create our own reality. And there are always two sides of everything, meaning that you can look at any situation as the cup is half empty or as the cup is half full. It is all a sense of perception. The empty signifies the negative side and the full signifies the positive side. So when you are looking at the full side you are focusing on the positive side and that is easy because you feel joy, but what do you when you witness something unwanted? My suggestion is that you look away and find something, anything, more joyful to focus on. The more you practice this the more you will attract more positive things, people and situations to come into your experience. This is what I like to think of as looking through rose colored glasses. I like to think about what I do want and not give much attention to unwanted things except to notice that they are unwanted. I then immediately shift my thinking to more pleasant thoughts even if it is something non-related to what I don't want. Eventually when I have my self in a good frame of mind I can think of the wanted in a more prosperous way.

For a while now that is exactly what I have been doing and to tell you the truth I have never been happier. I can see now why people experience whatever it is they are focused on. After 9/11 I found myself watching the news intently and I was becoming more and more scared to live in my own country. I was sinking into a deep depression and I knew I had to do something drastic before I became totally paralyzed by my fear.

The first thing I did was to stop watching the news. I couldn't take it anymore. They just kept talking about it in an endless loop and it got to be mind boggling. So as the days went on I found that by focusing on more pleasant things, like my children, I could feel joy enter my life once again. I truly believe that by this one act of looking away from unwanted truths I started finding my authentic self. And once I started down this path things started changing rapidly for me. And because I was being more selfish and caring more about how I was feeling about everything, things got a little hectic for a minute. I ended up leaving my husband just as the recession got started. Money got very tight and I could hardly pay rent. But I'll tell you I was much happier than I had been in a long time. And I had faith that things would get better because life goes in cycles and this was just a dip in this time interval.

A short while later my husband passed on to the next phase of life and I became a widow. This made it so that I could collect his social security and his pension. This helped for quite a while but the recession was still on going and I guess I was still buying into the idea that we should all be suffering. It took me a while but as I was sinking into the abyss I remembered that this was not who I am. I am not a (woe is me) kind of person. That's when I started looking for any way I could to raise my spirits. Instantly things started improving. Money started flowing more freely, my home situation improved, and my whole demeanor transformed for the better. I started reading everything I could find that would help me understand that I am truly the creator of my own reality, and I have the choice to see things, the way I want to, through rose colored glasses.

It has been a few years now and I am still on my beautiful path. So many wonderful things have happened and I know there is so much more to come. I have learned to see things in a much more loving way and I feel good 99.9% of the time. Keeping one's self happy is a full time job and I for one am willing to make that sacrifice. I know what it feels like to be depressed and don't wish that feeling on anybody. It is very true that it all starts on the inside. And once you get the hang of happiness you can't go back. *It just feels wrong.*

My son is in his twenties now and he has a very good job, government related, and he wants so much for me to hate the government the way he does. But what he doesn't understand is that by focusing on what he hates he is just perpetuating the unwanted and making himself miserable in the meantime. He asked me, "Why won't you hate the government with me mom?" I told him it is because I want to be happy. I feel that it is easy for people to look at situations they don't agree with and try to push them away, but all that does is make it bigger and more uncomfortable for the one pushing. We can't control what other's do but we can control how we react to it. What I mean is in order to feel better about a situation you need to look at the positive side of it, or the bright side so to speak. You know there are plenty of things the government does with our tax money that is really good. They build parks and highways for us to travel on. They also provide medi-cal for people that need medical attention and can't afford it. And don't forget food stamps for families in need of assistants. There are many more things like that for us to focus on, so you get the picture. I'm sure there are things that you could think of that you appreciate about the government.

In order to see things through rose colored glasses you must see things from the bright side. Sooth your anger, fear and hate by focusing on something pleasing to you and then look for positive aspects of what you are wanting, then watch and see how much happier you are and how your world is morphing right before your very eyes, just the way you want it to.

One thing we must always remember is that we can only control our own emotions. We cannot think, act or feel for another. Nor can any other think, act or do for us. We must all find our own way to happiness, and we must find a way of staying there as often as possible. Then and only then will we truly be the beings we are meant to be. Whoa! Did that hit you like it just hit me? I hope so because I really felt a jolt. So in essence what I got from this is that by staying happy I have the power to do, be or have anything I want to. And no one or anything can project any negativity on me that I do not desire. Keeping myself focused on what I do want, and staying happy on my journey to *whatever* that is, is all my work really is. I'm going to milk this feeling for a while. It is the most clear I have been in a long time. Not that I haven't been picking up nuggets of clarity all along the way. But once in a while you get a glimpse of something that just sums up all the answers to questions that have been looming in the background, and *BAM!, YOU KNOW!* You just know. Right now, what I know is, that life is good and I'm doing great, and wellbeing is abundant, and it just keeps getting better as I focus and stay happy, no matter what anyone else is doing. I choose me! And I hope for all your sakes you choose **YOU!** Live the life you want no matter what anyone else thinks. They can't think for you, only you know what is right for you. And that can't be wrong. And when you live this way things will always work out for you. Remember there is great love here for you.

Your loving friend,
Deb Mertan

MOMENTUM

have mentioned the word momentum in some of my blogs, but I really want to impress upon you how important momentum is. Have you ever had a great idea that just gave you goose bumps all over your entire body, only to lose the feeling after putting doubt on your path? Well the reason for this is that you are used to thinking that good things don't happen to people like you. You probably got a pretty good negative momentum going and it's very strong. Maybe you picked up the idea that things are not supposed to work out for you from a parent or a teacher, and it's been stuck in your mind all this time, or is it? What I mean by that is, that we all have the power to change our old beliefs or habits. You know that a belief is just a thought you keep thinking, don't you? And it only becomes a truth if you let it. So how do you change the direction of momentum? You start one step at a time. Even a thousand mile journey starts with the first step. It is possible, but it takes a willingness to think another thought until it becomes your new belief, therefore your new truth.

Now that I understand how the Law of Attraction works I can see why people are where they are in their lives. I can tell by the way they talk and by the results they achieve. This applies to good lives and bad lives. When someone is a complainer and acts like a victim they just keep attracting more of the same. It's just same results with different faces. If you haven't changed what's on the inside what happens on the outside can never really change, it's the law! It always knows what you are thinking and more importantly, what you are feeling. It's like when you are yelling at someone in an angry tone but saying, "Don't you know I love you?" There is a mixed message there because the feeling doesn't match the words.

So how do you get your momentum going in a positive direction? You pay attention. What I mean by this is you see how it feels when you say it

32

or do it, whatever it is. If it feels good then you are on the positive trail, but if it feels bad you need to re-direct your thoughts or words to match the good feeling. For example, if you are hating on someone, you are feeling bad as well. So in order to feel better about that person you either need to ignore them or try to find something about them that you like. It may take a few tries but that's okay too. After all, Rome wasn't built in a day, right? The more you practice finding good in other people the more good people you will find.

And another thing, you get what you expect to get. It's like when something bad happens and you say, "I knew that would happen." Well it happened because you expected it to. So why not start expecting good things to happen? It works both ways.

But sometimes momentum can be so intense that you just can't stop it. Unless, of course, you come to the realization that you are the only one with the power to do something about it. And there are those people that never do get it, like Jim Morrison of the rock band "The Doors." He had a destructive momentum going on. No matter how many people loved him and tried to help him he couldn't stop the drinking and drugs. Oh, he would try to stop, and it would last for a little while, but he would always return to drugs and alcohol. At one point he even went to jail for 4 months because he supposedly exposed his penis on stage, which was never proven, and used profanity. Of course he was clean when he got out, but that too was short lived. When someone keeps going back to the bad behavior it is because they have not taken the time to change their thinking pattern. They let what they see be their reality instead of creating their own reality. If they understood the Law of Attraction they would want to change the way they feel about everything.

Now I'll tell you a story about positive momentum, mine. Although my life is pretty amazing right now it hasn't always been. And even though I have always been a student of positivity, I didn't understand it the way I do now. It all started after my husband passed away. I felt like my life was falling apart and I couldn't seem to make ends meet. It seemed like I was crying every day and nothing was making any sense. So I actually sat myself down and had a long talk about getting back on track. The first thing I did was look for things on the internet that would help lift my spirits. I found some processes that really seemed to work and as I continued to look for new ways of feeling good, things miraculously started changing for me. It has only been 6 shorts years since that horrible time and I now own my own home. Believe me this has been one hell of a journey. In a good way. I went from almost being evicted to owning my home, what a ride. I have finally learned what it takes to make my life my own creation, and that is to keep myself happy and not try to fix anything, because there is nothing wrong or broken. At first the momentum was slow going but as I continue to practice feeling good and being happy things are moving much faster now. I love the feeling of inspiration I get as I trust that things are always working out for me. I not only believe that, I know it. Once you get to the place of knowing it just keeps getting better and better. I know that I am worthy, and I know that I am good and I know that I can have, do or be anything I choose. I know now that every time negative thoughts come to me all I need to do is stop the thought and find something else to focus on. Stop the doubt before it starts, so to speak. I pay attention to how I feel about everything. Have you ever heard the expression, "What would Jesus do?" Well here's a new way of saying that, "What would un-conditional love do?" When you start loving everything and everyone you will understand what I know to be true. When you let go of anger and judgement you release stress and hatred. When we are children we accept all others as equals. That is until we are taught to be hateful and judgmental. We all need to get back to that carefree time and stop worrying about what someone else is doing or not doing, and focus on what makes us happy. If we all did that we would all be living blissful lives. You think I'm kidding? I'm not, and you can bet on that. Words do not teach, but life experience does. All I'm saying is start really paying attention to how you feel about everything in your life. If you are going to a job every day that you hate you can't be feeling good. Or if you are in a relationship that is full of struggle that can't feel good either. So you have some choices to make in order to get back on the positive path. You can either, find something about that situation that pleases you, and focus on that, or you can start looking for what you really want and work toward that. Either way you will be moving in a direction and you can figure it out along the way. You'll know what feels good or not. This is the journey and that is the best part of all. If you look for the fun stuff and keep yourself in a good frame of mind you can't lose.

Now let's talk about un-conditional love a little more. You need to love yourself with that same mindset. It is important to be very kind to yourself and not beat yourself up over dumb things. Especially when you first start changing your beliefs. Whenever you have a relapse moment just laugh it off and eventually you will change the way you think and speak. It's a process, but one worth doing. And if you ever have any self-image concerns don't focus there. I'm sure there is something about yourself that you at least like, if not love. When you start focusing on the things you like the other things just start getting better too. You will be inspired to do something, like cut your hair in a stylish fashion. Or to buy some different cloths that feel friskier. These are just suggestions but I think you get the gist. If you allow it, your body will be whatever you want it to be. Again, it's the law. Remember, it's all an inside job. Your feelings are your navigational system and you should really listen to them if you want to live an awesomely happy life. And get that momentum going in a positive direction by feeling your way to joy. That's really all there is to this. It's not hard, but it is time consuming. In fact it is a whole new way of life. But once it becomes natural to you you'll know and you'll never go back the other way again.

So go on now and make yourself happy. It's the least you can do for the good of mankind. Live and let live and life will flourish right before your eyes. And always remember, there is great love here for you.

Your Friend,
Deb Mertan

ONE OF A KIND PAINTING

There is a new painting every day. Each morning as I drive to work and the sun is rising in the sky, I get the awesome pleasure of viewing the most miraculous scenes. The sky looks like a gigantic painting that changes continually, every second growing more and more vivid. Each time I look away and then look back at it I see a new painting. You know of course that we can't own these paintings, but that they are there for all to see and enjoy. They just keep moving and rearranging themselves to mesh with the beauty of the earth, showing us every crease in the mountains as the sun rises and the shadows fall where they may. And the colors blossom as the pinks and the greys and the blues blend with the greens and browns with specks of colorful wild flowers scattered randomly like sprinkles on a cupcake. The world begins to shine as the sun so intelligently rays down upon us to bring to our attention how abundant we really are. Abundance comes to us in many ways not just monetary gain. It's in everything around us. When you really think about it you could say, and really mean it, that we are abundant in oceans, and mountains, and sky, and birds, and trees, and friends, and family and so much more. I'm sure you as an individual can think of a lot more abundance in your life. When you start viewing life in this way, and realize that there is no ownership of any of it, it's on loan so to speak, and it is always here for all to appreciate. And by seeing everything with a cup half full attitude you will actually, greatly, positively relish your life. Now doesn't that sound delicious?

You know, when you stop clinging on to possessions and start sharing your things and talents the monetary abundance will naturally come. I know this sounds weird, but it is true. The more you don't cling to things and people the more things you want and people you love will flow into your life. Tricky eh? But once you try to own it or force it that's when things start to go south, and you end up losing out. What I mean is, hold on loosely but don't let go. If you cling too tightly you're going to lose control. That's a verse in a song and it always made a lot of sense to me. Have you ever had a mate that you loved so much that it hurt? And then it ended and your world turned upside down. It's like the earth opened up and swallowed you whole. That is because you were so dependent on that person to be your source of joy and happiness, and when you put that kind of pressure on another person it is bound to fail. But now think about a friend that you care about. You love this person but there is no pressure on the relationship because you understand that they are their own person and you accept them for who they are. You don't need them to do or act any certain way for you to love and appreciate them. And if for some reason you part ways it would be a little sad, or not, but it would not destroy your whole world. It's because you had no deep emotional attachment. When you treat everything with this attitude life will flow with ease.

If you really think about it life is always changing, second by second, just like the sky. We can't really hold onto anything. The most we can do is be appreciative while it is here and when it's gone think of it with fondness and be thankful for the part it played in this life that you created. Nothing is ever a waste of time because we always learn something new with each experience we have. Maybe if you start examining your life and see all the paintings that you have created you will find that it all fits together like a giant jig-saw puzzle. This painting connects to this painting then this one and so on. You'll see how all of it fits together to bring you to where you are now. Now is all we have so why not make it the best now you can? The more I live in my now the happier I get. My main goal is to be happy so when I look around at all the abundant beauty there is for me and all to see I feel very joyful.

I actually like to think of myself as a one of a kind painting. I am a constant changing canvas, and as the years go by I see myself improving with age. Every wrinkle and every line on my face reminds me of the wonderful life I have led. I'm not saying that I never had troubles or woes but I now see all of it as the journey that brought me to this place right now. It truly is the journey, not the destination that brings the joy we are all seeking. By the time I leave this world my whole body will tell the story of who I really am. The person I choose to be is a happy joyous loving caring being. And no matter how old I get I will be a great example of what an on purpose person is all about. I will paint the last and final painting of my life as a person that lived life to the fullest. And I won't be taking anything from this life with me. I will leave it all behind for someone else to use and enjoy. And once I pass through the veil that separates my human form from my infinitely intelligent spiritual form, I will never look back, but I will check-in every once in a while to see what's new. And I will smile down on my loved ones and send them all my love.

I really don't see why more people don't think like this. They save their money all their lives and hope that one day, maybe after they retire, they will be able to travel. But now is someday. Think about all the people that wait, and when the time comes to do all those things they were planning to do, they're too old or too sick to do any of it. Or the people that retire and don't have anything to do so they just die, never really have lived. Or what about the people that are born with some kind of medical problem and instead of trying to find a way to enjoy their lives they sit in a chair with a remote in their hand, watching life go by on television. They are so afraid of dying that they never really live. Life is supposed to be fun and adventurist and it can only happen for you if you let it. It's time to be brave and find your bliss and paint a new picture every day. It doesn't have to be some grandiose painting but it does have to be your own. The more you play with this idea the more fun you will have and the better life will be for you.

I guess I rambled on long enough for this one blog. There will be plenty more to come though. I hope you find what you are looking for and that this blog gave you a little boost to do just that. My only wish for all who are seeking their bliss is that they find it and milk it for all its worth. So that when you do leave this world you will have led the most awesome life you could ever think of. And what could be better than that?

Remember there is great love here for you.

With much love,
Deb Mertan

PMS, NOT WHAT YOU THINK

I know when people hear the acronym PMS they think of premenstrual-syndrome, and you can see why. PMS has been the curse of a lot of women, therefore their husbands and children, have suffered through it too. But that is not what this blog is all about. Yes the acronym is the same but I am giving it a whole new meaning. I am calling it pre-manifestational-syndrome. Let me explain. You know, if you have been reading my blogs, that I am a true believer of self-manifestation. And there is nothing we all can't be do or have as long as we focus on what we do want, and not on what we don't want. I'll use the analogy of the corn seed planted in the ground. You logically know that once the seed is planted that there is a process that could take weeks or even months that needs to occur before you'll see the full manifestation of the ears of corn on the stalk. If you were to get impatient and dig up the seed before it has a chance to grow you will kill the whole plan, dream or process. But if you wait patiently and watch for the signs of the corn coming, like the first sprigs of leaves poking through the ground, and then the little yellow balls that form just before they start forming into ears, and then voila', you can actually pick and eat them.

But wait, now you have no more corn. Oh dear, what to do now? Well if you really think about it we experience this similar scenario all the time. You see once you get what it is you are wanting it becomes old news. And yes it pleases you for a moment but then you find something else to go after. And if you are in this PMS state of mind eventually that will manifest as well. And once that shows up we are off to the next thing we want. It's when we try to force things to come that we kill the whole process. I guess kill is too strong a word, it's more like stifle. So the trick is to relax and let the Universe do its thing, because it knows what you want and knows

39

how to bring it to you. It is so fun to watch as all the components come together to bring you whatever you desire no matter what that may be. It will become a manifestation that not only you can see but others can as well. It's almost magic. And it is oh so fun when you watch for the signs and know that you are in sync with your desire, and then see it appear right before your very eyes. But it's not magic, it is the way it is supposed to be. And the only reason anybody wants anything is because they think it will make them happy. And since happiness is the goal, why not just be happy? Appreciate what you have and where you are in life and watch as it just keeps getting better and better. Once you get the idea to stop taking score of where you are and what you have or don't have, and realize that keeping yourself happy is the path to everything else you want, life will just seems so easy and fun.

Now let's talk about how to do this. As we all know there are plenty of things out there that can lead us down an ugly path. So how do you stay happy? By looking at something else that is more pleasing. When you focus on more pleasing things you will actually make it easier to find solutions to problems, rather than focusing on the problem, therefore perpetuating the difficulty. Nothing good ever comes from dwelling on the negative side of anything. As you can see there are two sides to everything. There is no dark without light, no good without bad, and no happy without knowing what sad really is. But once you experience the not wanted it is up to you to look away, bring yourself to a happy state of mind, then and only then, address the situation from a place of love and therefore bring a solution.

I know I've mentioned this in other blogs, but it bears re-iterating. What would unconditional love do? When we do everything from a place of love and appreciation life just flows more smoothly and we feel good most of the time. And when we have those rare moments of not so happy times we now know what to do about them, and we can bring ourselves back to a better frame of mind more swiftly.

So next time you hear the acronym PMS think about what you have been wanting and if you have been on the positive side or the negative side of it. You will know by the way you feel when you are thinking about it. And watch for the signs that are revealed to you all day every day that will lead you to wherever it is you want to be. Trust that the Universe is always communicating with you and is always on your side no matter what. But remember you will get what you think about whether it is bad or good. So go within and find that happy thought, let it gestate, and then move forward. Life is so good when you allow it to be. You are the boss of you so never forget that. Leave everyone else out of the equation when you are finding your bliss, and miraculously you will attract like-minded people into your realm, and life gets even better. Seriously when life seems like it's at its best it can get better, really! Believe me, I have been experiencing this for a while now, and just when I think life couldn't get any better, IT DOES! There is no limit in this infinite Universe. You are the only block of ANYTHING you want. You have all the magic inside you right now, if you only believe it and then know it. It's all up to you. Now no more excuses about why your life is not what you want it to be. Get happy and watch all the people and things that you desire fall into place just the way you want them to. This is not airy-fairy chit-chat. This is for real. I know because I am living proof. I am so happy right now and I know there is so much more to come. You can say I am excited about NOW and EAGAR for more. But Now is where its at and when the more comes it will be the Now of then. Its all happening now, and now and now, get it. Love who you are and where you're at and watch it grow like the corn stalk that brings you that ear of corn. Its so fun and liberating to stay happy and let others find their joy without judgement or condemnation. Live and let live is my motto.

So now you know what to do and what to watch for. Be kind to yourself. Don't get mad when you have an off day. Press the reset button before you sleep and wake up in a new frame of mind. Practice being your authentic self and life will be so amazing.

Remember there is great love here for you.

Your friend,
Deb Mertan

RE-TRAIN YOUR BRAIN

S o, if you have been following my blogs you know about the Law of Attraction. Therefore you also know that you get what you think about whether it's good or bad. What you focus on, even if it's for a short period of time, will become your experience. The law is always fair and consistent. It's like when you're dating a certain type of person and for some reason it doesn't work out, so you move on to the next person only to find the same person in a different body. And until you decide it's time to clean up your vibration, meaning your point of expectation, you will continue to attract that same person over and over again. When you realize this it is time to re-train your brain. It's not as hard as you might think. It just takes a little practice and some patients.

So let's say that you just broke up with your lover and you are feeling lost and alone. But that is because you are using that person as your source of happiness, and that's why you feel out of sorts and a little un-balanced. Now let's look at it another way. That person wasn't the right one for you. They were just another piece of the puzzle, letting you know what you don't want, therefore helping you figure out what you do want. And when you do look at the situation in this way you can actually feel the happiness grow inside you a little bit each day, until you realize that the happiness you were seeking was right there all along. This is you loving yourself more fully. And the more you do that the better you'll feel. When you are selfish enough to care about how you feel and you practice that often you will never go back to feeling down, at least not without knowing what to do about it. That's when its time to look for a new mate. But no matter if you date one person or a thousand people you are exploring and figuring out what is best for you. Isn't that nice to know. And each time you part ways with a potential mate you will understand that it is just part of the process and there is nothing wrong. In fact it couldn't be more right. Keeping yourself on an emotional high is the only way to live. This could seem a little tricky at first but once you get the hang of it you can create anything you want in your life. I like to think of it as my own little world. Each person is in their own little world. None of us thinks exactly alike. We all have our own ideas and our own feelings about what is right and what is wrong for ourselves. No one else can insert their feelings into another person. Oh they can influence another to manipulate them to do something, but eventually that will upset the relationship, and it will dissolve or fall apart. If you remember to live and let live and stop judging and condemning, and stop making anyone responsible for your happiness, life will be so fun. It is so important to know this because life can be whatever you want it to be as long as you take responsibility for your own joy. And let other people be responsible for theirs. The Universe is very tricky in that it can help every one of us have what we want without taking anything away from anyone else. It has a way of blending us all together in perfect harmony when we are in a happy state of mind.

I know that if you are new to this concept that it could be a little unsettling to think of being your own boss. But I promise you it will be very rewarding once you get into the rhythm of happiness, and you let it run to you and through you. It's like a stream that flows swiftly and you put your boat in the water and relax, the flow will carry you along with ease and you won't even need paddles. But if you were to turn the boat up-stream and start paddling it would be a very difficult struggle. You can tell which way you are going by the way you feel. If you feel good about what you are thinking, doing or who you're with then you are definitely going with the flow. So keep that in mind next time something up-sets you. Pay attention to all your feelings and gravitate toward the good ones and steer clear of the not so good ones. Just learn from them and move forward. That is how you re-train your brain.

Here's another example; Let's say you are working a job that you hate. Yes it pays the bills but it is not very rewarding. Every day you wake up with a grouchy attitude because you know you're going to have another crappy day. Things will never get better for you when you wake up expecting to have a bad day. So how do you change that? You start by focusing on something you can feel good about, even if it is not related to work, it will help to focus on that. You could try by telling yourself before you slumber at night that you will release all resistance about work, and when you wake up in the morning try thinking about how you want the day to go. You may only make it to breakfast before you think of something un-wanted, but that's okay, it takes practice. Just laugh it off and try again the next day. It will get better. As you keep doing this you will notice a change in the way you feel at work. And when you do feel better at work you might find that there are aspects of your job that you actually like, or you may find an opportunity to get a new job that you really love. But you must find your inner happiness first or you will just keep finding the same situation, just different faces and different places. It's like the guy that keeps doing the same thing over and over again, expecting different results. Or think of it like this, if you don't change what's on the inside, the outside can never change. Or you could say that if you don't change the vibration of your thought patterns you will just be taking yourself with you, and you'll end up in a loop of anguish.

You know it doesn't have to take too long to change to a different mindset. It's all up to you. The more you practice the faster it will change, and eventually it will become the norm for you to look for and find things that bring you joy.

And here's the last thing I'd like to mention. Whenever you want to start a project and you don't know how it's going to come or who will bring it or where the money will come from don't worry. Worry is not necessary. It only slows things down. Let the ideas come to you and relax your mind through meditation, or petting your cat, or taking a walk in nature. And when the inspiration hits you to make the next move then take action. The money will find its way to you. Keep thinking about why you want what you want, how it will make you feel and what about it will be fun. I promise you that when you approach anything in this manner all the components will be attracted to you. Just pay attention to how you feel and if you start to get a little overwhelmed take some deep breaths and remember to remember to go within, find a happy thought and bring yourself back to center. Think of it like this, the Universe knows what you want and knows how to bring it to you. That's how the Universe works. It may take you down some windy roads but when you look back you'll see that everything that happened was necessary to bring you to where you are now. Remember that you are the boss of you and you truly deserve all the happiness in the world. You don't need to wait until you're old to start traveling and getting all the goodies you have ever wanted. You just need to re-train your brain to know and believe that you can be, do or have anything you want. Think big and know that you are a very worthy being. Whether it's a lover a job or an invention, or anything else you desire, you can have it. All you have to do is figure out what you want and then let yourself have it. You know it's as easy to create a castle as it is to create a button. Life is good when you let it be, or should I say if you expect it to be. Remember to be your own boss and feel your way to bliss.

So are you feeling good yet? I think you are, or at the very least you're feeling better. Be kind to yourself and everyone else too. And remember there is great love here for you.

Your friend forever,
Deb Mertan

THINK BIG, THEN HUGE, THEN ENORMOUS

When I First started paying attention to how everything made me feel I realized that I had all the control of my emotions, and if I didn't like the way I was feeling I could just change it like a radio dial. It does take practice but it is well worth the effort. When I say effort I don't mean it's a chore or a job, but it is something that you must examine. I like to think of it as keeping up with myself as far as what I am wanting and what I am allowing myself to have. You see it all starts with you. When you figure out what you want and then you allow yourself to ponder it, to dream of it, to really feel what it would be like to have it, and then start to expect it, it has to come. The time it takes to get to you is really all up to you. How fast can you get yourself to that place in your mind, in your gut, to finally realize whatever it is you are wanting? The secret is to keep doubt, fear and fretting out of the equation because none of these emotions help anything. But if you get caught up in one or more of those yucky emotions, sometimes it's just best to let them run their course, crash and burn so to speak. Maybe go to sleep, or take a walk, or pet your cat. You see by taking your thoughts to a more neutral place you release resistance, which is what all those yucky feelings are, and get yourself back to a place of expecting once again. The more you practice the better you will get at it until the day that you know that all is right with your world and that is all that matters.

You know that dreaming of what you want is the beginning of everything on this planet. Not even a brick was made without someone dreaming it into existence. Now that might seem like a small dream, but as you can see that this small dream created an opening for a huge dream, like a building of some sort, maybe a castle, and eventually it became an enormous dream like the great wall of china, which took 20 years to build by the way. You see how that works. If you really think about it that's how thoughts work. You don't have to know how or when or who's going to bring it. You just have to be clear about what you want and let yourself imagine it, feel good about it, get excited about it and dream it into existence. The reason I called this blog, "Think Big, Then Huge, Then Enormous, is because it is easier to start with small things until you get the hang of the process and you start to notice things coming to you just by focusing on the positive aspects of what you want, why you want it and how fun it will be when it gets here. Inevitably you will start to dream bigger and when you really get the hang of it you will realize that there is nothing too big to attain.

I don't know if anyone has ever told you that it doesn't matter if you have a college education or if you only went to the 6th grade, you can still dream anything you want into existence. Do you know that Albert Einstein only went to the 6th grade and he is one of the smartest people to have lived on this planet? Granted there are people that really thrive in school and they just keep getting degree after degree but sometimes they don't accomplish much else. Haven't you known someone who went to college and after graduating they couldn't get a job, and they ended up working at a 7/11 store for minimum wage? So you see that it is all up to each individual to do what feels right to them. It's time to release all those old beliefs that certainly don't serve you and start new beliefs that make you feel good. You know that there is no shortage of goods in the world. You can have, be or do anything you wish without taking anything away from anyone else. Beliefs are just thoughts you keep thinking until they become your reality. We all live in our own little world and no one has the ability to push thoughts or beliefs into your world unless you let them. That's what weak minded people do but it doesn't have to be that way. Once you understand this concept and you become brave enough to control your own world, you will become so happy and so in love with life, that it won't matter how long it takes to be, do or have anything you want, because the only reason anyone wants anything is because they think it will make them happy. Happiness is the path to everything you want whether it's a mate or a business venture or a castle, it's all up to you and only you. And not everyone wants the same things. Some people are perfectly content with a simple life and some want it all. And of course there are all sorts of people in-between.

Another thing that I would like to mention is that it is never too late to start living the life you really want, or too early for that matter. Do you know that there have been kids that wrote books or started businesses or even invented something that changed the world for the better? And there are people well into their twilight years still discovering new things to surprise and delight them. The only thing that stops anyone from doing anything is a belief. Henry Ford said, "Whether you think you can, or you think you can't—you're right." Remember that song by the Rolling Stones that says, "Hey you get off of my cloud, don't hang around because twos a crowd." To me that means, "It's none of anyone's business what brings my bliss, so leave me alone." Joseph Campbell is another person that gave good advice, he said, "Follow your bliss." Wow, what a concept! I love following my bliss. I love being happy and not letting anyone or anything bring me down. Like Billy Joel says, "Keep it to yourself, this is my life, leave me alone."

So you see that there are signs all around us just waiting for us to catch the drift and remember why we are here in the first place. It's not to be perfect, because there is no such thing as perfect. And it's not to fix anything, because there is nothing broken. It's to live happily ever after. Really, I mean it. It's time to start listening to your inner voice and following the prompts that will lead you to the bliss you truly want and more importantly deserve. Actually your inner voice is more like blocks of thought or inspirational feelings that come to you. Haven't you ever found yourself going down a path you weren't planning to go only to find something you had been looking for but weren't sure how to find. Your inner being knew where to find it and because you let yourself follow the prompt you discovered it. This inspiration comes from our inner knowing but if you're not paying attention you may miss the clues. Think of it as a treasure hunt and every twist and turn is another clue to follow. It gets easier and easier when you pay attention. I'll give you an example of something I was wanting and how fast it came to me. I was listening to a podcast of a person that said that they kept $20 bills handy to pass out to homeless people. I thought to myself, I can't wait until I can give out $20 bills and it not phase me. Later that day I took a friend to lunch and when

I paid the bill I thought I was leaving the server a nine dollar tip, which I thought was good, but later I realized that I had left a nineteen dollar tip. I started laughing and told my friend the story of what had happened. I said, "See how fast the Universe delivers." Honestly it didn't faze me to hand out a tip like that. It actually made me happy to know that things could happen that fast. I know you've heard the saying, "Be careful what you wish for because it might come true." Well it should say, "It will come true." But if I had not been paying attention I could have missed that little nugget. There have been many more incidences like that in my life. You just need to be easy about what you want and let it come to you, and notice it when it does.

So now you know what's what and if you are wise, and I think you are, you will start paying attention to what you are thinking about and make good choices of what to ponder. Life is good when you believe it is so figure out what you want and let yourself have it. And remember there is great love here for you.

Love,
Deb Mertan

WEIRD LIKE ME

As I have evolved through my life I have come to the conclusion that the more different I am from other people the more I love me. I feel that the only way for anyone to be truly happy is to be who they really are. And the more you become the authentic you the more you will attract like-minded people into your life, and that's a good thing. What prompted me to write this blog was a conversation between my 10 year old great nephew and my 28 year old daughter. They were chatting about her new boyfriend, which is something she really likes talking about, and he told her that he couldn't wait for the weekend to be over so that he could get back to school to see his girlfriend. My daughter asked what was so special about this particular girl and he said, "Well, she is pretty and she's smart and she's weird like me." This just reminded me how profound children can be. We not only teach our children but they teach us all the time if we choose to take notice. I think babies come into this world already geared up and ready to do great and wonderful things these days. I mean 1 year olds are grabbing their mother's phones and going right to their favorite shows and actually watching them. I've seen it happen. But not only do we learn from our kids but through other adults that have thrown caution to the wind and said screw everyone else, I'm going to be who I really am, and if they don't like it, whomever they are, well that's just fine with me.

Let me give you some examples of the people I think are living or have lived their authentic life. One that comes to mind is Joan Rivers the comedian, she was a very courageous woman if you ask me. Being a woman in comedy was a rare thing when she started out. But she stayed true to who she really was no matter what anyone else said or thought about her. I heard her say in an interview early in her career that the secret to comedy is to tell the truth. Of course we embellish it a bit but that's what makes it funny. I have been dabbling in stand-up comedy a little and I have found that advice to be very helpful.

Another person I find interesting is Bill Gates. I can picture him as a teenager mastering his computer skills and coming up with new innovative ideas. And look at him now, he is a very rich and powerful person. But I'll bet he wasn't thinking about money, it was just the icing on the cake, oh yeah, a lot of icing.

Then there is Andy Warhol. That guy was way ahead of his time, but he intrigued people so much that even when he painted the Campbell's soup can everyone found it appealing. Apparently it is true that anything is possible.

I believe that all of these people had one thing in common and that is focus. They knew what they wanted and they put no doubt on the path. They found their inspiration and they followed the lighted trail. They weren't worried about how or when or who would bring whatever they wanted, they just kept moving forward until the magic started to lead them to the right place at the right time. And then they took action. Remember this is an attraction based Universe and when you try too hard to make things happen you usually get all balled up and nothing moves. But when you feel inspired to an idea it is always best to follow that nudge. Sure you can get a little ahead of yourself and things could seem to get a little squirrelly but that's when you take a step back and give your brain a break until the next inspiration comes. Or think about something else non-related to what you are doing and save yourself from the what-ifs. And you can't let other people bring you down either. When you have a good idea it's probably best to keep it to yourself until you really get a hold on it and your momentum is stable and sure.

There are so many others that have learned to tune out the peanut gallery, meaning all others, and do what makes them happy, with great success I might add. For instance Steve Jobs, Amy Schumer, Mike Myers, Adam Sandler, Tina Fey, Will Ferrell, the list could go on and on but I think you get what I mean. Even Albert Einstein followed his own path and lived the life he chose to live. We are not all meant to be the same so why not embrace your weirdness and live the life you want to live, and what's more deserve to live. Be your authentic self and let others do the same. Love unconditionally, and I mean everyone and everything and that includes yourself. Be ever so nice to yourself and eventually you will become the happiest person on earth and others will want to know your secret. Then you can tell them that you are loving more and criticizing less, especially about yourself, and that you are trusting that things are always working out for you. And that doubt, fear, worry and struggle are now taking a very back seat to joy, happiness, love and all other good feeling emotions so that you keep yourself vibrating at a very high level. If you just keep looking for things to feel good about you will slowly but surely only be looking for and finding those things and those people that truly match the frequency you are on. It's like tuning your radio dial to your favorite station. When you hear that sweet music that really turns you on you know you are there. And if you stay there more often your life will surely be a joyous adventure. You can't want too much because there is always plenty to go around. So think big, like the people I mentioned earlier. Don't let doubt take you down. Stop doubt before it starts by changing the direction of your thoughts and find something else that pleases you to think about.

I am so happy that my 10 year old great nephew is learning to embrace his weirdness at such a young age. I can see that he is destined for greatness in whatever he decides to do in his life. He has found the key to happiness and I hope he continues to find joy in all that he does. I hope that he will always march to his own beat and feel good and worthy all of his days here on earth and beyond. Just think how wonderful this world could be if we all just minded our own business and only concentrated on our own happiness, wow what a concept.

So are you getting it, that you are responsible for your own happiness, or not? You are the only one standing in your own way if life is not all you want it to be. You have to be happy before you reap any of the benefits you are after. Keep yourself on a high vibration and life will unfold before you in the most miraculous ways and eventually it will just seem normal for things to always work out for you. That is the way it is supposed to be. We knew before we were born and even just after that life was supposed to be good, but then other people tried to make us believe, through religion, government and school that we had to follow their rules and regulations if we were to be a "good person." But I see a change in a lot of people these days. This is a very exciting time when more and more people are realizing that they are the master of their own domain and that they have the power to be, do or have anything they want and not feel shame or guilt about it, because it's all good. We as humans are starting to get back to our roots, like nature, and we are now understanding the power of our minds and how connected we all are. We are all one spiritually and when we stop fussing and fretting we will not care what anyone else is doing or not doing. We will be free.

So now you know, you are supposed to be happy and life is supposed to be good no matter how weird you are. Now go out there and show the world what you are made of and don't worry about if they get you or not. They are just the peanut gallery, what do they know anyway?

Remember there is great love here for you.

Your Friend Forever,
Deb Mertan

WHAT DOES SATISFACTION FEEL LIKE?

S atisfaction is a word that doesn't get enough recognition as far as I'm concerned. What is satisfaction? For me it is a feeling of accomplishment, or a feeling of appreciation. When I feel satisfied I feel elation and love. To be in a state of joy is a feeling of satisfaction but sometimes it's hard to see how you could feel happy again. Especially when things that are totally out of your control occur in your experience. Then you might get a case of the what-ifs. That's when you second guess yourself or put yourself down in some way. But that's when you need to get into the practice of looking for things to feel good about. When a situation develops that you were not expecting, such as a break-up, it may seem hard to feel good. But even though you may not be able to find the best feeling to bring you out of your funk, you could find a slightly better feeling and as you keep practicing finding a little better feeling then another little better feeling you will eventually find yourself in a pretty good mood, therefore you will find the bad feelings have faded away into never-never land. Then you can focus on the things you really want to happen in your life. When you reach for better thoughts in increments it is a much easier path to get to the really good stuff that life is all about.

When you really think about it we never stop evolving. I'm sure you can think back to a time when you were much different than you are now. I'm also sure that it would be safe to say that over time you have been many different people and are still continuing to become a new and improved you. One thing I have come to understand in my own experience is that it is much more satisfying to not chase my dreams but to let them come to me naturally. I feel that when I am trying to make things happen the way I want them to, I get all twisted up inside. Overwhelming thoughts start to take over my mind and nothing seems to go right or make sense. When I have an idea I like to give it time to mature before I get started on the doing of it. I like to wait to be inspired to the best action, and then it feels like it is moving at the right pace at the right time.

You know, satisfaction doesn't have to be a big thing. It could be as small as a butterfly flying past you or a song on the radio that gets your juices flowing. When you really start looking for things that bring a smile to your face things will just flow smoother. I like to go around my house and look at all that I have accomplished up until now and just feel good about everything. I say things like, I love my kitchen and I love my floors and I love my windows, and even though it may seem silly to most people, what is actually happening is I am raising my positive vibration to meet my expectations of what I still want to come into my life. When you find appreciation in all the things that are current in your now, you make room for all the new stuff coming into your future. And if you really think about it there is never a future because when it gets here it is the now. Tricky huh? So staying satisfied is essential to living a blessed and happy life. People, you are never going to find happiness in a state of, I'll be happy when I accomplish this or when I acquire that or find the right mate. It starts with you and only you. When you figure out what it is you really want and then let yourself dream it and let it grow within you, nothing and no one else will matter. Yes it is wonderful to have friends and mates but they are not essential to your happiness.

I have been practicing these ideas for a while now and believe me when I say my life feels magical. Things that I would have never thought could happen have happened and life just keeps getting better and better. Loving life is a satisfaction all it's own. Once I started being deliberate about what I was thinking and how I was feeling everything went from doom and gloom to sunshine and lolly pops. I gave up worrying because it just didn't feel good and it got me nowhere. And fear was just as useless. When you are in a state of fear you become stagnant. All negative emotions are just indicators of what track you are on. If you are joyous then things can move forward, but when you feel sad or mad or blameful or any number of ugly feeling you stop all momentum. Is this making sense to you? I hope it is because it doesn't get any clearer than this. Stay happy, move forward, stay unhappy, stop movement.

So where do you want to be? What do you really want? And what are you going to do about it? These are questions you should be asking yourself on a daily basis. Keep yourself on your toes and then see what miracles await you. In fact after you start witnessing these so called miracles you will come to know them as truths and they will seems normal and natural. I know I've said it before but I'm going to say it again and again, Life is supposed to be good. If you need to remind yourself of this very important fact put sticky notes up anywhere and everywhere to keep it in your face. Do whatever it takes to keep yourself as happy as possible, and when you find yourself a little unhappy change the subject to a topic that is better for you at that moment. It might be a good idea to have a list of things that make you happy to look at when things are a little off. If one thing doesn't work try something else. Different moods call for different actions, but only you will know what is best for you.

I could go on and on about this all day but until you start practicing being happy and seeing the good that comes from it my words are just words. It's like your mom giving you good advice but you think, what does she know? Then what she warned you about happens and you say, oh damn, she was right. But you had to see for yourself, right? Well this is the same thing. It's up to you to do it or don't do it but either way it is your choice and it's okay. This is your life to live any way you want to, happy or sad. Everything is a choice and we all live in our own little world. We are our own master of creation and we can be, do or have ANYTHING we want to. When I say ANYTHING I mean it. Don't sell yourself short. You don't have to be the smartest person on earth or even the most popular person, you just need to be the best you that you can be and that is good enough. Never listen to the peanut gallery. Those are just people trying to get you to do want they want to make their selves happy through you. You are not here to please anyone but you. In fact when you are trying to please everyone else you please no one, especially not you.

So, what have you learned here today? If you read it right you should have learned one very important thing and that is to stay happy at all costs. Unless you enjoy being miserable, that's up to you, and that's perfectly alright too. But if I were you I would go for the gold. Be the shiny beautiful soul that you are meant to be and love yourself with all your heart. You will be so glad you did. Remember that there is great love here for you and wellbeing abounds. So until we meet again.

With all my Love,
Deb Mertan

WHAT'S THE RUSH?

In this day and age things seem to always be so rushed. Or at least that is the way I used to feel about time in general. There never seemed to be enough of it. I always felt that I was running around doing a million things at once and really never accomplishing anything in a significant way. Sure I got things done like laundry and dishes and regular everyday tasks. I always felt very organized but at the end of the day I was too tired to do any of the things I had always dreamed of doing, because there was no time. But like most people I thought this was perfectly normal. It wasn't until I was much older and I became so overwhelmed in my everyday life that I started looking for ways to make myself feel better. That's all I wanted was to just feel better, not good or fantastic because that was just too big of a leap. That's when I started looking on the internet to find any way of making myself feel better. I found positive quotes, little exercises that you work at every day, and mantras that when repeated were supposed to bring your spirits up. Once I started utilizing these methods I was led to other ways of finding joy. They came in the form of books, articles, CD's and even the Oprah Winfrey show. I really started paying attention to all the good things that were happening because of my new attitude and it was awesome! That's also when I learned about the Law of Attraction and realized that it was real, and I was actually bringing everything I wanted into my life.

Now that I was aware of what was happening and that I was in control of my own feelings, I was noticing how time seemed to slow down and I could do so much more in the same amount of hours that I had thought to be too short. Even traffic seemed to be lighter when I drove on the freeways. I never seemed to be late to anywhere I had to be. It seemed that the slower I went the more time had. I stopped feeling that angst about having to hurry for any reason. Haven't you ever seen someone on the road weaving in and out of traffic trying to get ahead of everyone else? Only to pull up to the red light and they are right next to you. All that rushing around really did no good. If they had just stayed calm and went with the flow of traffic they would have had a much better trip.

Another thing I noticed is that things were coming to me as I was ready for them. It's like you wouldn't want everything you're going to eat in your life to come all at once. You want to savor each meal and enjoy the taste and texture, swirl it around in your mouth and relish every bite. That is how I feel about everything now. I want to adore all there is to see and do and experience. Life is so good when you slow down and let it come to you in increments. Have you ever heard the saying, "Stop and smell the roses"? Well that is what it means. Stop and look around at this beautiful planet and really see the beauty. People sometimes get so busy that they never even pay attention to the sunset. They forget that life is supposed to be fun, and they get so twirled up in what they have to do that they keep their head down and their nose to the grind stone, and that's not fun.

As humans we sometimes make things harder on ourselves than need be. What causes this is the belief that we need to please others rather than ourselves. When we try to please everyone we end up pleasing no one, especially ourselves. It's time for all of us to start being more selfish about how we feel, and if it don't feel good don't do it. It is time to understand that you and only you can change your whole world.

Let's talk about other things we as humans might be in a rush about. Like romance for instants. I know that the idea of being in love is beautiful, and we are all seeking it in some way or another. But when we just hook up with someone because we want a relationship so badly that we just settle for the first person who comes along, it doesn't always pan out the way we would like it to. I'm not saying that love at first sight doesn't ever happen because I have met people that knew they had found their right mate right away, but that is rare. What I am saying is that when we're out in the dating world we should take our time and figure out what we really want before we make a full on commitment. Like I said, "What's the rush?" If you go into a relationship with no expectations or pre conceived ideas of what the other person should or should not do and just let it unfold naturally you will be able to relax and have fun, no matter if that is the right one or not.

There are so many people in this world so why not give a few of them a try and see how they fit for you. In the mean time you can figure out what works and what doesn't work. It's all relative and only you will know what fits best for you.

If you give it some thought can't you see that rushing really gets you nowhere? There is so much to see and do along your path of life. The journey is the only thing that matters. Once you get whatever it is you are after it will only thrill you for a moment and then you are going to be off on the next excursion to find something new to do or have. It will never end because life in infinite and so are we.

It's time to learn how to chill and get back to basics. There are so many ways to relax and have fun. Heck even laying in the grass and staring at the clouds can be fun. I love to see how many animals I can find in the clouds as they slowly drift by and change right before my very eyes. The simplest things can bring such joy. Even just sitting on the front porch with a cup of coffee, watching the sun set is exhilarating to me. Time is precious and so are you. It is so important to take care of yourself because you are the only one who can. It is not anyone else's job to make you happy, nor is it yours to make anyone else happy. Yes it's nice to be nice to others but not at the expense of your own happiness. Now is the time to look for ways to invigorate yourself and live life to the fullest. Once you start finding things to make yourself happy you will see that everything you want will unfold for you. The trick is to stay happy as much as you possibly can and life will be so good. Worry and fret will be a thing of the past and joy will replace all the ugly feelings that have plagued you. Life is supposed to be good, fun, joyful, happy, and exciting and any other word you can think of that means alive.

So there you have it. You know now that there is no rush. Time will flow so smoothly once you let go of the angst that causes stress and worry. You really can create your own magical world once you slow down and take time to smell the roses. And always remember there is great love here for you.

Love,
Deb Mertan

YOU'RE ALWAYS HERE, YOU'RE NEVER THERE

I once had a boyfriend that always said, "I'm always here, I'm never there." At the time I didn't think too much about it. But today as I was driving to work the idea popped into my head that this statement was very profound. It is the truest statement I have ever heard. If you really give it some thought you can see that it makes a lot of sense to those of us who are always striving to live in the now. If I am always here then I must be living in the now. Just like there is no tomorrow, because when tomorrow gets here it is actually today. Oh yes, you can think about tomorrow or the future but you are doing it now. And you can travel to there, but once you get there you are actually here once again. When you pay attention to where you are it is a much happier way to live. You don't need to justify how you got here, only know that everything that has occurred in your life has brought you to this point in time and it is exactly where you are supposed to be. And you don't want to think too far into the future because the what-ifs start popping up and you can get crossways of what you are wanting.

Life is supposed to be fun. Sure, there are things that we do that most people would consider not fun but if you really look for it there is an element of fun in everything we do. Half of the fun is looking for it and finding it. People spend too much time fretting over things they have no control over and that is what gets them all balled up. The only thing we have total control over, if we choose to practice it, is our emotions. Think about the animals of our world. They do not fret, not one little bit. Especially our domestic pets. They are not worried about getting up on time for work or what they are going to wear today. They don't ask what's for dinner, they just wait until the bowl is full and then they eat what's there. They have no doubt that they will be taken care of. We need to feel more like that in order to free up our minds to think about more fun stuff to do.

Or think about it this way. What if you were a new born baby? You don't worry that you will starve. You give a little cry out to mom or dad and they come with a bottle. And when your diaper is dirty they change you. And besides sleeping those are the only things that you need. Life is simple and good. If you really stretch your imagination you can see that this is how the Universe works. When you start believing that everything is always taken care of for you, you can relax and enjoy yourself. Use your emotions as your guide. The happier you are the more things will go your way. Once you practice this for a while you will never want to go back to fretting. You will realize what a waste of time it is and how bad it is on your wellbeing. You must realize that happiness is a choice and once you apply it to your everyday life you will feel better. Not only emotionally but physically as well. I have said this before in many of my blogs that everything starts on the inside. That means that the only way to feel better is to fill yourself with happy thoughts and be as loving as possible. When you choose to share your love and joy you attract other like-minded people and it becomes a constant loop of bliss. Why would anyone want anything less than that?

One thing that works well for me is to smile at myself in the mirror, and say, "I love you Deb." When you love yourself fully you see it reflected back through the eyes and actions of others. It gets more and more exciting to me to see how loved I am through others. And it also reflects back from our domestic animals. They just seem to gravitate to me now in a way I have never known before. It makes me know that I am on my right track and I have nothing but great things in store for me. It is so easy for me to talk to people and play and have fun in everything I do. I look for the right person to sit next to on an airplane or at the lunch counter in a restaurant. When I purposely sit next to someone it always turns out to be a fun time. You may be thinking that you are too shy or embarrassed to talk to a stranger but believe me it is more fun than you think. You're probably never going to see that person again so who cares if you act silly. In fact being silly is what children do all the time and they don't worry if someone is looking at them funny. Have you ever watched a young child at a doctor's office playing and laughing, while all the adults are somber and serious? That's because they know that there is nothing serious going on here. They are a great example of always being here. If I were you I would stop worrying and fretting, and I would kick fear to the curb. Life is so good when you let it be. Give yourself permission to be free and take deep breaths when you feel overwhelmed. Line up with your inner being and see how great things really are. Treat yourself the way you want to be treated and you will see that others treat you that way too.

I love my life so much that I can't help but share what I have learned with all of you lovely people. And once you start filling yourself with this everlasting joy you will want to share it too. It becomes addicting and then contagious. But it is better than any drug that is out there. It is a high that will become a euphoric familiarity that you will want to cherish forever. Remember there is nothing serious going on here and you can't get it wrong and you'll never get it done. New thoughts and ideas will constantly be coming to you and life will continue to get better and better.

So what are we talking about here? We are talking about being present in the here and now and staying as happy as possible. Making better choices and look for the fun in life. How much easier could it be? Be happy, be happy, be happy! And then be happy some more! Okay so now you got it. So go do it. Practice fun, joy and love. Life will change in what seems to be in miraculous ways, but in reality that is the way it is supposed to be. And one more thing, remember there is always great love here for you.

Forever, Your Friend,
Deb Mertan

YOU BE YOU, AND I'LL BE ME

I have been practicing being in alignment with my inner being lately. What I have realized is that the more attention I give to myself, the more I have no time to worry about what anyone else is doing. This is actually a feeling of great freedom. It may seem selfish, and for sure it is, but this is how I came to the deeper understanding of what being true to yourself really means. The trick is, you really have to mean it and practice it until it becomes a natural way of life.

What some might not understand is that by being true to yourself first and foremost, you can be of much more benefit to yourself as well as others. It's like the flight attendant on the airplane says to you," Put on you oxygen mask before you help anyone else." That's because if you pass out while trying to help others no one will be saved.

When I finally decided that, you be you, and I'll be me, I realized that I was actually allowing myself to be who I wanted to be without the worry of what anyone else was thinking of me. It's like the fortune cookie I got once said, "Dance like no one is watching". And now I can recognize those others that feel the same way. In fact I feel that I am attracting them like a magnet. I love that it doesn't matter to me what anyone else is doing in their lives. We are all in our own little world and life is supposed to be fun. Of course we can make our world any size we want to, it doesn't have to be little.

Now that I have given myself permission to live the way I want to time seems to be moving at just the right pace. I have plenty of time to do all the things I want to, and it seems like everything schedules itself perfectly so that I just follow the lead to where the best stuff is. I know now that it is not my job to make anyone else happy. My only concern is how I feel. When I keep myself happy I am not infringing on any one and in fact I am bringing a bit of joy to everyone I encounter. But of course it is everyone else's responsibly to keep their selves in a joyous state.

If everyone would take care and pay attention to their own feelings the world would be a much happier place. I know a couple that were very happy together, but eventually they started growing apart. One of them was feeling very uncertain about where things were going and wanted to break it off. The other one was devastated of course but there was nothing more to discuss. It was over. But during the next 8 months they both started really getting to know their selves again. They realized that they were both up each other's butts all the time and really lost who they once were. When they finally did work things out they realized that they had different interests than each other and that it was okay. In fact it was more than okay, it was liberating. They realized that loving each other was enough and that living in each moment was so much easier than trying to look too far into the future. They even stopped complaining to each other about stuff that really didn't matter. They found that it was much easier to communicate in a positive way, which takes the stress out of the equation and lets the good stuff flow in.

You can't help but be who you are. I have a friend that grew up in a time when being gay was very taboo. He played the role of straight man for quite a while. He dated girls in school and eventually married and had 4 children. But after 10 years of marriage he finally broke and decided to come out of the closet, as they say, and all hell broke loose. His parents were disappointed to say the least and his wife was appalled. His kids were scared and confused and friends didn't know what to think. Naturally things settled down and eventually it seemed normal when he finally got to be who he really was.

I actually fell in love with a man that is not yet ready for what I have to offer. He may never be ready. Like I said I can't worry about what anyone else is doing or not doing. After going through all the whys and what fors, and trying to stop seeing him, I again gave myself permission to love him no matter what. I realized that he has lived a very different life than I have and that he is working on his own self. As much as I tried not to love him so deeply I had no choice. My heart knows what it wants. We still see each other from time to time but instead of worrying about how much I don't see him, I thoroughly enjoy our time together. I know he loves me too but

I also know that when you try to force things to happen the way you want them to things get mighty ugly. So some day we may become a couple but for now we are very good friends and you can't get enough of those.

So if you haven't gotten the gist of what this blog is all about, it's like this, just keep your nose out of everyone else's business and care exponentially about your own feelings. Keep yourself on as happy a thought as you can in each moment of the day. At first it may feel strange to you but that is because you have been so used to complaining about things you have no control over. It's time to start thinking about what you do want, not about what you don't want. And when you have a dream or desire to be, do or have anything, be nice to yourself and let yourself have it. And stop beating up on yourself when you think something has gone wrong. You can't get it wrong and you'll never get it done. If you're doing it right life will just keep getting better and better and you will never run out of things to want. Like I said, life is supposed to be fun so get out there and find it. It just takes practice, so what else have you got to do?

Now that you know what to do I hope you start doing it. Like right now! No one else can do it for you. Give yourself permission to feel good and you'll see your world change right before your very eyes. There is great love here for you. And your inner being will always be with you, loving you, assisting you, having fun with you, showing you, knowing you, guiding you, and the list goes on and on. Follow your bliss and you won't go wrong.

With all my love,
Deb Mertan

DO UNTO OTHERS

Have you ever thought about how other people treat you and why? Like when you are in a bad mood you seem to run into other bad mooders. (I just made that word up, but it fits, doesn't it?) And when you're in a really good mood you run into really fun people. Well the answer is in the question. Whatever you are projecting out you are receiving or attracting back. So when you want to be treated a certain way you should project it by treating others the way you want to be treated. That's where that saying comes from, "Do Unto Others as You Want Others to do Unto You." It makes sense doesn't it? This is also known as the Law of Attraction. This is the only law that is relevant when it comes to living a life that you, and only you, choose. People are always blaming others for their bad moods or misfortunes. But the truth of the matter is we create our own reality whether we realize it or not. You see your mood is your indicator of how you are projecting and what is coming to you or what you are attracting. When this becomes clear to you, you will want to pay closer attention to your moods. It will become very apparent that when you feel bad you just can't catch a break. And when you feel good things just seem to work out effortlessly. It's true but only you can figure it out for yourself.

Words don't teach, only life experiences do. I can tell you things all day long, but until you see it for yourself it won't matter. And the way you do that is by paying attention to how you feel and what you are thinking about, and what is manifesting around you.

Other sayings that are used quite often are, "Like attracts Like" and "That which is Liken to itself is drawn." Sometimes we don't realize that we are attracting something until it feels like it's too late to change it. It happens so gradually that we don't see what has manifested until we are knee deep in the problem or situation and we feel stuck. We can always change the situation but it doesn't come through action. We need to first do the mental work.

Let's talk about a person who has found their self in a toxic relationship. I'm sure you know someone like this or maybe it's you. This person has met a partner and at first the relationship is going pretty well. They date for a while and then decide to get married. The honeymoon is wonderful and their life is good. But one day the bottom drops out, so to speak. One of them becomes angry for something that seems silly. The other one brushes it off as a onetime event. But weeks later it happens again. Now the other one is getting a little worried about this behavior and starts getting nervous around them. Then other people notice that this person is not as perky as they used to be. They ask questions but the abused person always says, "Oh it's nothing or I'm fine, just tired", or something to that effect in order to keep the peace at home. But as time passes this person becomes more secluded and sadder. Maybe it has been years and they feel beat down and scared to move on. What should they do? Well the first thing to do is start treating their self the way they want to be treated and deserve to be treated. When they have a good day or even a good few moments, they should milk it for all it's worth. And when it is a bad day keep reminding their self that they are a worthy joyous being and that being happy is a state of mind. And the next time something good happens milk it for all it's worth. That means to try to stay in that feeling for as long as you can. When you start changing on the inside you will see things on the outside getting better and better. When you love you things have to get better, it's the law.

Now it won't change overnight and you might get a little worried about that, but don't, that will only slow you down. Just find things to be happy about even something as small as hearing a bird sing in a tree. Anything that makes your heart sing is a good thing. Pay attention to your emotions because you get what you think about and what you feel about. Eventually you will teeter to the side of the scale that is mostly happy and you can move on if you so desire. You actually have to give yourself permission to be happy. And again you have to milk it for all it's worth for as long as you can. And each time you do this it will last a little longer until happiness is normal for you. You should never feel guilt or shame because it is our right as humans to feel good. That is what all of us want and we all deserve it.

And it all starts on the inside. We need to love ourselves first and foremost no matter what else is going on around us. We need to pay attention to our feelings and not let anyone else try to control how we feel. Not a mate or a parent or a teacher or preacher of any kind can guide you as well as you can guide you. You are unique and that is a good thing.

I know that it may seem hard at first to change how you feel, but believe me if you keep practicing it will happen. It did for me. I have not always been this happy, but now that I am I don't let anyone or anything bring me down. Oh I have my moments but they are short lived. I know how good it feels to feel good, and when I don't it's just not tolerable anymore. I don't like being angry or scared or worried. I gave all that up because I know it's just a waste of time. Solutions come to a clear mind. So I meditate and appreciate and I treat people the way I want to be treated.

Now you know what to do. I hope you do it. You are the only one who can. Be nice to yourself and others will be nice to you.

And as Abraham always says, "There is great love here for you."

Sincerely,
Deb Mertan

GOD IS COLORLESS

Do you know why I call my web site "Love Equals Love"? It's because I want to convey the message that what you put out will surely come back to you. And most of the time it's a lot better than you could have imagined. Life is supposed to be good and when it isn't it's up to you to figure out what it is you truly want. The way to do that is to sift and sort through life and when things happen that you don't like, that will let you know what you really want. But it would be very hard to jump all the way from not wanted to wanted. It has to come in increments. Little by little you will figure out how to turn a negative into a positive. It takes trust that what you want is coming and that who you are is worthy of all that is. This is also what I have come to think of as true freedom. Once you understand that you are the creator of your own world and you start leaning it that direction things will slowly but surely start lining up to bring you all the things you dream about. Whether it be a big pile of money or a lover or a dream job, it doesn't matter, if you want it, it will come. It has to come. You need to give yourself a break when changing the direction of your life. After all it took a whole lifetime to develop the beliefs you have. But you need to stop and ask yourself "Are these beliefs serving me to my best advantage?" If it feels good then the answer is yes, but if it doesn't feel good then the answer is no. And it would be in your best interest to change to thoughts that make you feel better. Just a little better will get the ball rolling and as you keep looking for better and better thoughts eventually you will see evidence of what you desire coming to you. When you really get the hang of catching yourself in the midst of an uncomfortable thought you will notice it and change it much more swiftly.

Seriously I am not just making up little stories to make people think that they can change their lives without firsthand knowledge of what I am saying. I have been practicing being happy for a few years now and my life has changed dramatically. I mean I was getting evicted from a rental when I first started and not only did I not get evicted but I actually bought a house a couple of years later. It has been an awesome journey and it just keeps getting better and better.

I'm going to be perfectly honest with you right now. I have been writing blogs and giving you different processes by which you too can change your life and live your authentic dreams. I use words like momentum and re-train your brain and inspiration, but what you may not realize is that I actually do these processes I write about. These are not just words, these are guides in a sense. These words are meant to help you to remember to remember what you are here for. And that is to have fun and to love for the sake of loving.

Let me tell you what you can expect when you practice being happy all the time. You will get a whole new perspective of life and people and even animals. Especially animals. They just seem to know that you are in a high frequency vibration and they want to be around you. And I don't just mean domestic animals, I mean Birds and lizards and even snails. I know it sounds weird but that's what's happening. Then time slows down. I never feel rushed and I'm always on time to anywhere I go. And it seems like I have a lot more time in the day then I used to have. And my timing is right on, whether I'm telling a joke or just saying the right thing at the right time. And writing blogs is becoming easier and more prophetic. I just seem to be smarter for some reason. And when I say I want something it seems like the Universe goes out of it's way to line up all the components that will help bring whatever it is to me. It's like things just fall into my lap as soon as I decide I want them. It's almost miraculous, and I say almost because I'm now understanding that this is the way it is supposed to be. This is what normal is and I mean for everyone, not just me. Life is supposed to be good, we just have to remember how loved and worthy we really are. And it can only come from one place. It starts with you and only you. You have to be the one that decides you want to be happy no matter what. So arguing with someone will be a thing of the past. It won't be important to be right anymore if it takes away from your happiness. And good people will flock to you as well. They will want to know your secret of joy. And you can say, "I am joyful because I care about how I feel.

I use my emotions as my GPS guide. It doesn't bother me that someone is a different color than I am or that they live a different life style than I choose. I don't worry about who thinks what. And if any of that mattered don't you think God or whomever you believe in would have made us all the same color?" Maybe we would all be like robots and do everything the same if that were the case. So God must either be colorless or He/She is very multi colored. So I just go with the flow and let life live me. I ask for what I want and then relax in the knowing that it is on it's way. I don't need to know the details of how when or who is going to bring it. And I only take action when I am inspired to do so. Even writing these blogs has to come from a powerful urge to get up and do it now.

Here is an example of a powerful urge. I went to the garlic festival in Gilroy Ca. and after I parked the car my friends and I went to the trunk where our luggage was located and put on our sunblock. It was a very hot sunny day. Then we proceeded to the bus that would takes us to the fairground. All of a sudden I got a very strong urge to go back to the car for a bottle of water. I felt like I had completely dried out and I had to go back. When I turned to go to my car I saw that the trunk was wide open. I knew without a doubt that I was being led back to the car so I could close the trunk. I truly believe that the Universe or God or the source of energy that flows through us and everything on this planet always has my back. And if I pay attention to the signs and nudges and follow my bliss life can only get better.

My advice to anyone who wants it is to be easier on yourself. Take more naps. Pet your cat more often. Be playful and stop worrying about anything. Worry doesn't serve you in any way except for a brief moment to remind you that you are a little off track. It's like that little voice inside you saying, "Oh yeah, I don't need to do that anymore, I do this now." Then you can smile and say with full knowledge that there is nothing serious going on here. Life is supposed to be good and it's okay to love everyone even if they are different than me. And once you get the hang of being happy everything you want will find it's way to you. It's like planting a seed in the ground. You put it there knowing that with some tender loving care it will grow into whatever plant you put there. You're not going to plant corn and then see a rose bush come up. Have faith that whatever you ask for will come if you just keep nurturing the idea of it and let it come naturally, and the better you get at it the faster things will come.

So be off with you, now. Go forth and smile. Be playful and have more fun. Be silly as much as possible. Jump for joy and stop and literally smell the roses. Life is what you and only you make of it. And you CAN be do or have anything big or small, it's all the same as long as you believe. And remember there is so much love here for you.

Forever and always,
Deb Mertan

SHIT HAPPENS!

As some of you might know I have a lot of roommates. I am a single woman with a four bedroom house and I rent out all the rooms to people I know and love. But just because I know and love them doesn't mean they will always get along. And most of the time they do, but recently we have had an upset. There is a new guy here and no one seems to like him very much. He has been my friend for about ten years and I like him a lot. But for some reason one of the women I live with accused him of taking $100.00 out of her purse. Now normally this would be cause for quick action, but for some reason I wanted to wait to talk to him. Part of the reason was that the holidays were among us and I didn't want an up roar during a time that is supposed to be joyful. And also I didn't want to believe that this person would do something like that. And when I did talk to him I wanted to be prepared with a plan of action. As you know I am a firm believer in keeping myself in a good mood. I wanted to confront him when I was calm and filled with love in my heart. Of course the woman that told me about this didn't want me to wait to talk to him, so I told her that she could confront him if she wanted to. She decided to wait for me to do it.

Thanksgiving arrived and we all had dinner together. It really went well. We had lots of other guests and after dinner we played games and ate pie. It was lovely. The next week after Thanksgiving we all went to Georgia to watch my son graduate with his master's degree at Georgia Tech. Of course I didn't want to ruin that either.

When we got back home I decided to at least confront him to see what he might say. Of course he denied it. He even went to the woman and told her that he would never do something like that but that he understood that because he was the new guy it was logical that she would think it was him. Now everyone in the house knew about the incident. That's when one of the other women in the house said that she too was missing $100.00. Now things were looking bad for my friend. Everyone wanted him out. But I kept my cool because I have been practicing keeping calm for a while now and I know that getting upset doesn't help. I trusted that the Universe would work this out and that somehow it would all end on a happy note.

So now Christmas arrived and all our guests came to party again. My daughter came with her boyfriend and was telling us about the house they are living in. she said that they had recently found out that the people they were living with were doing meth. This made them very unhappy. I told her that they could come live with me but that it would have to be in the living room with a partition. But she had one more month of school and the drive would be too much for them. And they really needed a private room anyway. Everyone in the house heard her story, including the new guy. But that was the end of it for the time being.

Later that week my daughter called me and asked about our situation with the new guy. At that point I had not made any decisions but this gave me the perfect opportunity to tell him that I needed the room for her. But again I didn't want to ruin any bodies holiday so I waited until New Year's Day. There was also one other little thing that needed addressing, and that was that he was having trouble keeping up with the rent. So this gave me a good place to start our conversation. I sat him down and said, I'm sorry to tell you this but I need to take the room back for my daughter. And besides you haven't been up on the rent and I really depend on that money. That's how I pay for my house. I need everyone to pay their share. He said he knew this was coming because he heard the conversation at Christmas. I told him he had a month to find a place and he was grateful for that. He totally understood and we even hugged and told each other we loved one another.

You see this could have been an ugly thing but I refuse to get myself all worked up anymore. It's not worth it. I know things are always working out for me, and all of us actually. We just need to stay happy as much as possible.

Now I know it may seem that I was being insensitive to my other roommates that felt violated, but that was not the case. I needed to keep myself in a good frame of mind so that when I did talk to him things would just go smooth and there would be no anger involved. I couldn't prove one way or the other that it was him and neither could they. And I also know that when you let the Universe take care of things it will always show you the path of least resistance. And it all worked out as I expected it would. People also have to realize that when shit does happen it is because of what they are vibrating. They are broadcasting a signal into the Universe and they are literally attracting what they are getting. When bad things happen it's not the Universe picking on you. You are bringing it even if you don't know you are. You have to be aware of what you are focused on and what is coming to you. The Universe doesn't hear yes or no. It only sees what you give your attention to and brings you more of it. So if you are focused on something you like and you don't put any doubt in your way the Universe will say, oh you like that here's some more. But if you are saying no to something the Universe only sees that you have your attention there and says, oh here's more of that as well. It's up to each of us to pay attention to how we feel and what is coming to us as a result. So it is very important not to let anything bring you down.

When you are feeling sad or mad or any other ugly feeling it is because you are not in agreement with your inner being. Your inner being is always looking forward and looking on the bright side. It's light hearted and loving everyone and everything. When you aren't it feels bad. But when you are happy and feeling frisky you are in alignment with your inner self and you feel joyful and invincible. What I'm trying to get across to you is that you can't hold anyone else responsible for how you feel. Even when shit happens you have to take responsibility for your part in it. Pay attention to where you are vibrating. When you start taking responsibility for everything that comes to you it will be easier to change your vibe and climb up the emotional ladder, so to speak. You have to feel good where you are now. And as Abraham-Hicks says, it's okay if it's just a small improvement because that's all you can do, but it's enough because that's all you can do, but it's enough. You see you will get a little bit better each day and before you know it you will be happy most of the time. And things will be good most of the time. Then when shit happens again after you have been keeping yourself in a good mood, which is also being in alignment with your inner being, it won't seem as dramatic. And you will be willing to wait for the right moment to act. You see the contrast or shit that we have lived through is what has helped us know what we don't want so that we can focus on what we do want. We need to lean more in the direction of what we do want so that things like people steeling from us is a thing of the past. Really, you have more control over your life than you realize. And now is the time to realize that you and only you can make the change. And when you do tip the scale toward everything is always working out for me, you will say, it happened because I asked for it and I want some more please.

I know this is going to sound weird but it is important to appreciate everything and everyone, even the bad stuff. Sometimes the Universe takes you to things you want in what seems to be bad ways, but it actually ends up being good. I know that we have all had things happen that later after thinking about it we realize that if that didn't happen this good thing couldn't have come.

When all the stuff started happening in my house I had to hold fast to my beliefs and not get all caught up in the problem. I had to let the solution come to me and it did. You can't focus on the problem and the solution at the same time. You acknowledge the problem then quickly turn your attention to the solution. And once you turn you need to trust that the answer will come and that everything will work out. Your higher self is always with you and always has your back.

These are the things you must stop if you want to live an exceptional life. Stop worrying. It does no good to worry. It accomplishes nothing. Stop struggling. When you struggle you just go deeper into the problem, like quick sand. Don't hate. It only comes back to you in really ugly ways.

Here's what to do to feel good and live the best life ever. Stay happy as much as possible. It feels so good to be joyful. Play more. Playing is one of the best ways to raise your vibration. Laugh as often as possible. Laughing is a great way to fill yourself with joy and release any unwanted negativity. Love more. I mean love the trees and the flowers and the birds and the people all around you. Just love. And most of all appreciate. Appreciate the beautiful day or the rainy day. Appreciate the food you eat and the people that grow the food. Just appreciate everything and everyone. Everything that you have lived has brought you to this place right here right now. Now is all there is so make it as good as possible.

Look, you are not going change your habits and beliefs over night, but if you start now to see which habits and beliefs serve you and which don't you will start feeling better bit by bit each day. You have to do the work though. You have to look for ways to keep yourself happy, and in a short while you will see everything morph into a life with more joy and love than you could have ever imagined. It's not hard but it is different than what you have been used to. But believe me it's worth it.

Now get out there and show the world through your actions how it's done. Show yourself how you want to live your life. Show the Universe that you trust that everything is always working out for you.

Remember there is always great love for you here.

Sincerely,
Deb Mertan

TAKE WHAT YOU WANT
AND LEAVE THE REST

I n this day and age information is rampant. I mean that if you want to know about any subject all you have to do is ask Google and 50 thousand ideas will pop up for you to explore. It can be overwhelming. And there are a lot of different opinions about every subject. So how do you decide what is good for you? How do you decide what will work in your experience when there are so many ways to do something or see something? It comes from perspective. Perspective is everything. And when it comes to you, your perspective is the only one that counts. When you read something or watch a video on any subject you are the only one that knows how it feels to you. That is your perspective.

I personally love to read. And I have my favorite authors, but sometimes I like to see what someone else has to say. But if it doesn't resonate with me, or if it doesn't feel good, I just leave it alone. I choose to believe what I believe and I don't let what doesn't feel good bother me. And I don't try to force my ideas or opinions on others. I believe in the idea of live and let live. I can't and don't want to think for anyone else. My life is enough to take care of. And I feel I'm doing a great job of it. I pick and choose from all the information out there and when it feels good I know it's right for me.

I truly love my life but it wasn't always so. I had to figure out who I am and let myself be me. It can be hard when you are trying to please someone else or live up to some impossible standards. I know parents that try to make their kids be something they don't really want to be. Like a father that wants his son to be a football player. Maybe the son wants to be in band or be in drama class. But when he tells his dad he wants to do something else the dad belittles him, and makes him feel like he can't make his own decisions. It happens all the time.

I actually knew a boy that was in drama class. I gave him a ride home one day and he told me that his dad was very disappointed in him, because he thought of acting as being gay or for stupid people. But I happen to know that this boy is very talented and very smart and handsome as well. He had it all and he did it well. But the dad wouldn't even come to his plays to see how wonderful he was. But the good part is he never veered from his dream and now he is an actor. He knew what felt right to him. Yes, it was hurtful when his dad didn't come to see what he was doing, but in the long run the dad gave in and now he sees how wonderful his son really is.

So what I'm really trying to say here is that you need to be true to you first and foremost. You need to be who you really are if you want to live a happy life. And isn't that what we all want, to be happy? So when you are reading or listening to someone about how life should be, take what feels good and leave the rest. Only you can know what feels right for you. A belief is just a thought you keep thinking until it feels true. So think thoughts that really ring true and make them your new beliefs. Pay attention to how it makes you feel and you'll know if it's right for you. Everyone is different and that is a good thing.

Now go do what's right for you and love your life. Give yourself permission to be happy and see how life morphs into the best life ever.

Remember there is always great love here for you.

Your Friend,
Deb Mertan

TELL A NEW STORY

I feel that most people believe that they have to live the life they have been dealt. Maybe they grew up poor and always heard things like, "Life is hard", or "Money doesn't grow on trees". So they go through life not expecting it to be any different. But I'm here to tell you that it doesn't have to be that way. It's time to take back your power and tell a new story. Start by deciding that you can be do or have anything you desire for your life. Did you get that? You can only decide for yourself, not anyone else. That's important to remember. And yes, it is that easy to turn in the direction you want to be heading. But it takes practice, and as you know anything worth doing does take practice. You know, like driving a car or using a computer or flying a plane. Whatever you fancy takes practice.

As soon as you decide to believe that you can be do or have anything you desire you can start talking about how you want your life to be. The best way to start is by being general in your statements about your new life. Example: Let's say you are wanting more money to flow into your reality. You could say something like, "There is plenty of money in this world and I know I can have as much as I want". This is a very general statement that you could believe. And as you keep saying or even thinking about this you start to feel it in your body and it becomes a new belief, which is literally just a thought you keep thinking over and over again, until it feels real to you. Once you feel it you can start saying things like, "I know my money is on its way and things are always working out for me". Then you can start thinking about how you will spend your money and how much fun it will bring.

Here's a good example from an actual friend of mine telling a new story. She lived in Ohio her whole life. One day she decided that she wanted to live in California. So for about 3 months she kept telling anyone that would listen that she was moving to California. No one believed her but she knew that it would happen. She didn't know when where or who would help it happen, she just knew it was going to happen. Then one day she got a phone call from a friend she knew as a child that lived in California. Her friend said that there was a room available in the house she was living in and it was hers if she wanted it. You see, she never doubted it for a minute, and viloa, here she is.

Now let me explain how this happened so fast for her. It was because she never got too specific at first about the details of how, when or who was going to bring it about. As she kept saying and thinking about this move she started to get rid of things she would not be taking with her and packing things that she would be taking. This was a little more specific as she let herself imagine and feel what it would be like to be in California. And that was all that was required for her to see how the Universe will bring what you want in life as long as you don't doubt yourself or the Universe.

So after getting the phone call to go to California she invited a friend to drive out with her and they essentially made a very nice vacation out of it. They even went to Disneyland before she actually moved in. They had a very good time all along the way.

Wayne Dyer wrote a book called, "You'll see it when you believe it". That is one of the truest statements I ever heard. It is how children see things all the time. The little ones haven't been trained out of their ability to dream, imagine and believe that they can be, do or have anything they desire.

Have you ever met a chronic liar? You know they're lying but you can tell that they are really believing their own lie. That is because they are telling the story so often that it feels like the truth to them. Sort of the way our politicians act these days. You could argue with that person until you are blue in the face and they won't budge.

So what does this tell you? It's saying that if you want to change something in your life at first it might seem like a lie or a fantasy. But if you keep talking in general terms, like my friend did about California, and you keep saying it until it feels real to you then the specifics will fill in for you and you will see for yourself how the Universe is always fair and consistent. You get what you think about, period! It really does feel like magic at first but once you really get the hang of it you will see that this is normal. Life is supposed to be good for everyone. We all make our own choices. We all have our own dreams. And if we don't let anyone talk us out of those dreams they will manifest. It's all up to you and how well you tell the story. (Maybe just keep it to yourself until you feel pretty good about it.) And once you feel good about it you will start to believe it, until you come to the point that you know it, because you will be living it.

You know, the Universe or God or whomever you believe in is always with you. Just because you can't see it with your eyes does not mean it does not exist. Most people grew up in some sort of religious background where there was a God figure. Did you see that God? NO! You just trusted that God was hovering around watching and judging you as you went through your life, trying to live up to some impossible standards that some church or government or teacher told you would help you get into heaven. If you think about it, the Universe is the same thing. It's an invisible source of energy that is always ready and willing to bring to you anything your heart desires. But in this scenario there is no judgment. We are meant to be, do or have anything and everything we want. And once you get what you think you want and it doesn't feel right anymore you have the right to change your mind. This is called re-inventing yourself. It just takes trust that you, the human you, is in concert with the spiritual you, and together anything is possible. Like Wayne Dyer says, impossible is just saying I'm possible, after you break it down.

So this is my suggestion to all who are not living the life they want and to those who are but just want to boost it up a notch. Dream, imagine, smile more often, look for reasons to be happy, ignore the nay sayers, look for ways to have fun, be funny, love yourself more and more, and believe me you will see it come back to you. Just like the infinity sign, what goes around comes around. Your life can be whatever you want it to be no matter where you are now. That's just the starting line. So on your mark, get set, GO! You're ready to be your authentic self. Don't worry that the others in your life aren't ready for you. Either they will catch up or go away, it's all good.

Remember there is tremendous love here for you.

Sincerely,
Deb Mertan

TODAY IS SOMEDAY

How many times have you thought, someday I'm going to blah, blah, blah, only to save a few bucks and then something happens where you have to spend the money for some kind of emergency or car repair, or you get the picture. Then you start over and it happens again. You never get ahead because you are always waiting for that someday. Well that is a rut that's hard to get out of unless you know about the Law of Attraction. When you are always living in the future and you are waiting for the perfect opportunity to go somewhere or buy something or even have a baby you are not living in the now. Now is where someday is. Now is all we really have. Yes even if you are thinking about the past or looking toward the future you are doing it now. And when you learn how to be present in your now things will start changing for you. I know I've said this many times but it is still true that each and every one of us is creating our own individual world. We CAN be, do or have anything we desire. We just need to chill out and let our desires come to us by thinking what and why we want it. But when you have to explain why you want it by complaining how bad it is without it you are not going to get very far.

There are always two sides to your desires so when you say, I want to buy a new car, but I don't know how I'm going to get it, you just shot yourself in the foot, so to speak. But If you say I want a new car and it's going to be great, and I'm going to have so much fun driving it, and people will say, oh man you have a great car, you start filling yourself up with the positive energy that the Universe will pick up on and will go to all sorts of lengths to bring it to you.

I probably told this story before but it is a really good example of how the Universe will go out of its way to bring you what you want. I was driving my Chevy Cobalt that had been in a wreck. I didn't have the money to fix it because at the time it happened I needed to catch up on bills, so I used the insurance money for that. But the car still drove okay so I Just kept driving it. After a few years of driving around like that I started thinking about how nice it would be to have a new car, or at least a newer car. But I really didn't have the money for a down payment and I was still paying on this car so I just let that thought go for a while. But I kept appreciating that I had a car at all. And then I started collecting data about what I would want in my next car, like power windows and Bluetooth capabilities. And I would like a bigger car like an SUV. But I wasn't in a panic over it. I would just see things in other cars that I liked and say, oh I like that feature. And wouldn't that be nice? And I would appreciate all the new technology. And all the time I would still keep appreciating my old car for all the years it served me.

Then one day without any warning my car just stopped running. I just coasted over to the curb and called a tow truck to take me to my mechanics shop. I figured he would be able to fix it and I would be back on the road in no time. But later that day he called me and said I had blown a rod and I needed a whole new motor. Well I could have gotten upset but I didn't. I just said I didn't want to replace an engine on a car that old so I would just look for a used car in the meantime. He said he had a car that he would sell me for $1500.00. I said okay but I would have to make payments. He agreed and I picked up the car the next day. But this was probably the worst car on earth. It smelled like gas because it had a leak, and the locks were all corroded, it only had two doors and it was a stick shift. It just sucked all the way around. So as I was driving it I just casually said, I really need to come up with a down payment for a newer car. As I was coming down an off ramp I looked over to see a sign that said, Grand re-opening Mazda dealer, $88.00 drives you off the lot. I thought, Wow I could do that. So later that day I went to the Mazda dealer and sure enough the sign was correct. The salesman asked me what I was looking for and I said I want an SUV. He pointed to one that had just come in. I walked around it and said I'll take it. He asked if I wanted to test drive it first. I said okay but in my mind it was already mine. When we got back he checked my credit score and said I qualified. But I didn't have all my paper work with me so I told him I would be back in the morning. The next day happened to be Mother's Day so my son came to visit me. I asked him to take me to the dealership and within two hours I was driving off the lot with only $88.00 down. How often does that happen? And because I only had the sucky car for a week my mechanic took it back and returned my money. That whole incident showed me that I could do anything. The new car even had all the technology I had been asking for and I didn't even realize it until I had been driving it for a few days. All of a sudden I realized that everything I had been putting into my daydreams about a new car came true. It just all happened so fast that it didn't register in my mind right away.

This is where paying attention comes in. Because you could be dreaming about something you want for a while and putting details in the dream as you go along, and as long as you don't doubt it or put your dream down in any way, it has to come to you. But because it came gradually you might have forgotten that this is exactly what you have been asking for. So when you do feel like something good has come to you think about what you have been focused on and see if you can remember putting all the pieces together to bring you whatever it is you have been asking for. The more you realize that you are the creator of your own reality, the more you will realize that the Universe is always working for you. But you must also realize that when you focus on unwanted things the Universe will bring that too. That's why it's important to pay attention to your thoughts because they will manifest good or bad. Remember the saying, "Be careful what you wish for because it might come true"? Well change that to, "Be careful what you wish for because it WILL come true."

There are ways of getting better thoughts going through your mind. One is to look for things that bring a smile to your face. Like smelling roses or seeing a flock of birds flying in sync. Or holding a new born baby. Whatever makes you smile is okay with the Universe. And when you start looking for things that make you happy the Universe will go out of its way to show you more things like it. And Vise-versa. It will always reflect back to you whatever you are focused upon. The Universe is always fair and consistent. But don't get upset if you happen to get off on a tangent of something unwanted. That just lets you know that your guidance is working, because if you know what you don't want it helps you to know better what you do want. Life is supposed to be fun. It's really all up to you. When you live in the now you will notice how everything you want will morph its way into your existence. No matter what anybody else is doing or not doing doesn't matter. You are you and you can be, do or have whatever it is you want.

Another way to start living in the present is to chill out more. Relax and let life flow through you. When you stop worrying about how, when and who is going to bring what you want it will come easily. But all those negative emotions just slow it down or stop it completely. That's when people say, "I feel stuck". They aren't stuck. They are just focused on unwanted things and the always consistent Universe will just keep bringing those same kinds of things. Different faces, different places, but same stuff over and over again.

And the last thing I'm going to mention is if you want to really get things moving in the direction you are wanting, start appreciating everything and everyone, even things and people you think are bad because those things help you get perspective and gain knowledge of what you really want. Its all good.

So now you know that you are the master of your own domain. And you are a powerful being. And life is what you make of it. And always remember there is great love here for you.

Sincerely,
Deb Mertan

WASH, RINSE, REPEAT

No, I'm not talking about shampoo. I'm talking about life. Have you ever known someone who just keeps doing the same thing over and over again and they keep getting the same results. You know this is what's considered to be a crazy person. They just keep doing the same thing expecting different results. Yes the results may vary slightly but in essence it's the same thing.

Let's break this down so you can really get the picture. So I know this guy that has been married 4 times. The first time was when he was about 19 years old. He had two kids with her but she was very jealous and had a habit of hitting him. He never hit her back because men are taught to not hit girls at a very young age. But some do, I suppose. But he didn't and one day he just ended the marriage. Then he met a woman with a couple of kids and he moved in with her. Then she decided not to work anymore and he ended up supporting her and her kids. So he ended that relationship. He then married a cute thin woman who really liked sex. He thought he struck gold until she decided she didn't need to take care of herself anymore and gained about 50 pounds and stopped liking sex. So again he ended that relationship. Then he met another woman who seemed to really like sex and she made her own money and for quite a while it seemed that he had finally got it right. But eventually she became hooked on prescription drugs after several back surgeries. He really tried to stick it out for as long as he could but when she started to threaten to kill him in his sleep he decided it was time to go. At this point he swore he would never get married again and then just a few short months after his divorce was final he did it again. This time to a woman that controls him through self-pity and threats of suicide if he leaves her. Do you see a pattern here? He has a momentum going that just keeps repeating over and over again.

Now let's break down the title of this blog. WASH- this is the fun part. Like when you put the shampoo in your hair and you swish it all around until the bubbles are flying everywhere. But then you have enough of this because the bubbles die down and it isn't fun anymore. RINSE- this is the break-up. You rinse the shampoo out until you are squeaky clean once again, like a clean slate. But you really haven't cleaned up your vibration so that you can find the new feelings that will help you get out of the rut you are in. So what happens is, you REPEAT- the process. There's nothing wrong with that if that's what you want or if you are liking what is going on. But I don't think that he was enjoying all that. The point I'm making with this story is that this man did not give himself any time at all between women to figure out what he really wanted. He was still caught up in the same beliefs and habits that kept bringing the same types of women to him. It's true that you get what you think about. So if he were to start thinking about what he wanted in a relationship and really given it some real airtime by imagining and day dreaming and desiring, he would have started a new momentum through new beliefs that would have served him much better. He just didn't stay single long enough to know who he really is and what he truly wants.

This sort of behavior is very common amongst the human race. But I truly believe that people are waking up and figuring out that they have more control over their lives than ever before. We are no longer under the influence of our parents or our government or even the church people. We are becoming more aware of our emotions and using them as a guide to know what feels right and what feels wrong for our individual desires. Not any two of us want exactly the same things, and that is a wonderful thing. And just because we want something different doesn't mean that it's wrong for someone else to do what makes them happy. Even if it's your spouse or any other person you deal with on a regular basis. The Universe or God or whomever you believe in will make it so that everyone gets what they want and blends us together so that we can all be happy. The key word here is happy. To keep yourself happy means you don't give a rip about what anyone else is doing, and don't worry that someone else doesn't like what you're doing. No one else can feel for you. Only you know what's right for you. And once you get comfortable with your new feelings and new beliefs and new habits it will get easier and easier to be your authentic self.

I know I say this a lot, but here it goes again, LIFE IS SUPPOSED TO BE GOOD. It's okay to be selfish in the respect of doing what feels good to you. Nothing is off limits. Oh you may think that there are people out there doing things like killing or stealing, but they are not happy people. They do those things out of being disconnected from their authentic self. But if you are truly happy it is okay to be do or have anything your little heart desires. And just because some stuffy old person says that it is bad to have sex or to drink or to smoke or whatever society says is wrong or inappropriate does not mean they are right. They are the ones that make all the dumb rules and laws to try and keep the masses under control. But only you know if you are inappropriate. And if you ask me I would say, be who you are and never mind the rest. Be gay if you're gay, be sexual if it suits your fancy be funny and silly if it makes you happy. Like I said nothing is off limits.

So what's the gist of this blog? It's to wash, rinse and not repeat if it feels off to you. But if it feels good do it again. Only you will know. So go out there and be you. The world is going to love you just the way you are once you love you. So until next time remember there is tremendous love here for you.

Forever and Always,
Deb Mertan

WHAT TO EXPECT WHEN YOU LOVE YOU

Self-love is at the basis of being your authentic self. But for most of us it has been taken away at an early age by people trying to guide us by what they were told and by what they lived. People like parents and teachers and even government who want us to please them. But the only problem with that is that those people are fickle and they keep changing the rules so it makes it impossible to please any of them. And in turn no one is pleased, especially not you. I like to use the analogy of the flight attendant. They tell you that if the oxygen masks fall to put yours on first before you try to help anyone else, because if you can't breathe what good will you be to anyone else? It's time to take your power back and learn a whole new set of rules. Your own rules. Those rules that let you be who you really are. The rules that you and only you set for yourself. You can't expect anyone else to make you happy either. It's like when you have a partner that is mostly always pleasing, someone that makes your heart sing whenever you're around them. But sometimes they may be in a bad mood or just grouchy or just down right tired. But if you are keeping to your true and authentic self and letting happiness come first that person can't bring you down. They can't inject their bad mood on you unless you allow them to. When you are aware that you have control of your emotions, and you choose to be happy no matter what, you will be on your best path ever. Believe me, I've been there and now I'm here where life is good and I can and do choose to be joyful no matter what else is happening around me. I'm not saying that you or I will never feel bad again. I'm saying that you or I will be able to recognize what is happening earlier and get back on course faster.

Do you know what self-love really is? It is being nice to yourself. It is caring about how you feel. It is loving who you are right here and now even if you aren't where you want to be just yet. It is being happy whether you are in a crowd of a million people or all alone. It is taking more time to relax and daydream and exploring what you really want out of life. It is re-inventing yourself over and over again because life keeps moving and you need to keep up with it. And it's not beating up on yourself when things do get a little out of hand. It's okay to feel a little bad sometimes because that just helps guide you to what you really want. This is normal because we are humans and we have feelings that help guide us to where we really want to be. This is literally the only control we have as humans. We can't think or feel for anyone else but ourselves. And when you discover this for yourself life will be as good as you let it be.

Now let's talk about an easy way to get to know yourself fully. My personal favorite way to get clear about what I want and who I want to be is to meditate. Meditation used to sound like something mystical or weird even. But now day's people are really embracing it, and realizing what a great tool it is for getting ready for the day. Setting the mood so to speak. It is a great way to relax and put everything into perspective. Here is an example of how I do it, but believe me there are many methods to choose from if mine doesn't work for you. This is what I do most every morning. I wake up and get myself some coffee then I use the bathroom and make sure I'm ready to relax with no interruptions. Then I sit in my recliner and set a timer for 15 minutes. I close my eyes and relax. I count 3 breaths in and 5 breaths out which helps me not think too specifically about anything. I let the thoughts come and go as they will. It sort of feels like my mind is sorting my thoughts into the right files, like organizing. Then when the timer goes off I feel refreshed and ready for the day. Sometimes an idea will pop into my head right away and I'll be inspired to do something or call someone or an answer to a question will come about something I've been wondering about. And sometimes I just feel so good that I go through my day looking for and finding all sorts of things to be happy and appreciative of. Which in turn makes my whole day a wonderful experience. Only you will know when you start to feel the relief of stress and worry through this process. And if my way doesn't work for you there are hundreds of meditation CD's for you to choose from. It's all good. Just remember that as long as you keep trying you will eventually get to the place of true self love. And after that anything is possible. It takes practice, and I mean all day every day. You will eventually reach a tipping point where you will no longer be willing to feel bad, at least not for very long. You will use your bad mood as an indicator that you need to change your train of thought to get back to the good feelings again.

So you see that self-love is the most important love there is. It is the only way to truly be happy. And after all what else could be more delicious than that? Now get on that super wave length and show the world what a happy person can do. You know what I'm talking about. Get out there and be the you, you were meant to be. And don't worry about anybody else. They are none of your business anyway. And you aren't theirs either. And when someone tries to bring you down tell them that you've tipped in a new direction and if they ever get there you will see them on the flip side. Because you are too busy being happy.

Just as a reminder, there is always great love here for you.

Your True Friend,
Deb Mertan

YOU'RE TRYING TOO HARD

As many of you might know I have been making it a habit of staying calm, and letting life unfold for me. What I mean by that is that I am enjoying my journey. I try to make sure every day is as fun and frisky as possible. I love interacting with other people, especially strangers. It seems like everywhere I go I meet fun people to play with. You never know what kind of fun can come your way. I have come to the point that I expect that the day will turn out to be fun. It's all perspective. Fun can be anything. Even doing dishes can be joyful if you let it be. Putting the dishes in the dishwasher can be like putting a puzzle together. I like to see how much I can get in there as neatly as possible. Fun doesn't have to be bouncing off the walls enthusiasm. It just needs to be pleasing to you.

Let's talk about a situation where someone is trying too hard to make something happen. Like a woman trying to get pregnant. She keeps an eye on her menstrual cycle and tries to have sex on the right day at the right time. But month after month no baby. So she and her husband go through all sorts of tests and procedures, but still no baby. The desperation sets in and what happens after that, they give up. Yes they stop trying and sometimes they go so far as to adopt a baby. Then what happens is they get pregnant, because they are not focused on getting pregnant.

That's just one example but it doesn't only happen with babies. It happens all day every day. People want something so badly that it almost hurts. But once they stop trying to make it happen it comes, like magic. But it's not magic, it's the way it is supposed to be. You have to let it come, expect it to come and enjoy the path to it.

I know there have been things in your life that you briefly thought about and then all of a sudden it pops into your life. That's because you had no resistance to it. You weren't trying to make it come to. You just casually let it float through your mind and didn't doubt it, and it came.

Listen, Life is supposed to be good for all of us. Whether we want to be rich or just satisfied with our lives, it's all good. We don't all want the same things out of life and that's perfectly perfect. But the one thing I know for sure is that we all want to be happy. And happiness comes from within. You have to be happy first to bring more happy things and situations to you. Once you get in the grove and you fill yourself with joy you will see all sorts of things change in your life.

Here are some of the things I notice in my life that have changed for the better. First thing is I am never rushed anymore. Even when I'm driving I don't feel I have to hurry. And when other cars speed by me it doesn't get me nervous or scared. I know they have control of their vehicle and I have control of mine. And another thing is how animals like me a lot now. I have never been an animal person per say. I don't hate them I just never wanted any of my own. But since I have been keeping myself happy animals have been gravitating to me. People tell me how their dog or cat never likes anybody, but they like me. That's because animals can sense pure joy and that's what they are all about. And the next thing is how people treat me now. I'm sure that when I am out and about people can sense my vibrational premise as we meet, and it shows from the smiles and hellos I get. The biggest smiles come from the little ones. I love to interact with babies. And I never worry about money either. I know that when I need it, it will come. I trust that the Universe always has my back. I know now that I am on my right path because I feel good most of the time. And on those rare occasions that I don't feel good I just ride it out. I do things like pet the cat or dog. Or I take a nap. And when I go to bed at night I tell myself that all resistance will subside while I sleep and in the morning I can start with a clean slate. I can feel any way I want to so I choose to feel happy.

This is something that takes practice. It won't happen overnight. It will come in increments. But the more you practice the better you'll get at it. It is a life style change. And once you see for yourself how you can change your life to be as happy as mine, you'll want to keep doing it. Happy has nothing to do with people places or things, it has to do with you loving you. And you are more than you see in the mirror. You are a spiritual being having a human experience. You are pure love. And when you realize that you can share it with the world. And life will be whatever you want it to be. I promise!

Remember there is always great love here for you.

Sincerely,
Deb Mertan

LOOKING THROUGH ROSE COLORED GLASSES

I know most people think that they need to look at what is and react to it whether it is something wanted or something unwanted. But the truth is that we all have a choice to react in any manner we desire. We honestly do create our own reality. And there are always two sides of everything, meaning that you can look at any situation as the cup is half empty or as the cup is half full. It is all a sense of perception. The empty signifies the negative side and the full signifies the positive side. So when you are looking at the full side you are focusing on the positive side and that is easy because you feel joy, but what do you do when you witness something unwanted? My suggestion is that you look away and find something, anything, more joyful to focus on. The more you practice this, the more you will attract more positive things, people and situations to come into your experience. This is what I like to think of as looking through rose colored glasses. I like to think about what I do want and not give much attention to unwanted things except to notice that they are unwanted. I then immediately shift my thinking to more pleasant thoughts even if it is something non-related to what I don't want. Eventually when I have myself in a good frame of mind I can think of the wanted in a more prosperous way.

For a while now that is exactly what I have been doing and to tell you the truth I have never been happier. I can see now why people experience whatever it is they are focused on. After 9/11 I found myself watching the news intently and I was becoming more and more scared to live in my own country. I was sinking into a deep depression and I knew I had to do something drastic before I became totally paralyzed by my fear.

The first thing I did was to stop watching the news. I couldn't take it anymore. They just kept talking about it in an endless loop and it got to be mind boggling. So as the days went on I found that by focusing on more pleasant things, like my children, I could feel joy enter my life once again. I truly believe that by this one act of looking away from unwanted truths I started finding my authentic self. And once I started down this path things started changing rapidly for me. And because I was being more selfish and caring more about how I was feeling about everything, things got a little hectic for a minute. I ended up leaving my husband just as the recession got started. Money got very tight and I could hardly pay rent. But I'll tell you I was much happier than I had been in a long time. And I had faith that things would get better because life goes in cycles and this was just a dip in this time interval.

A short while later my husband passed on to the next phase of life and I became a widow. This made it so that I could collect his social security and his pension. This helped for quite a while but the recession was still on going and I guess I was still buying into the idea that we should all be suffering. It took me a while but as I was sinking into the abyss I remembered that this was not who I am. I am not a (woe is me) kind of person. That's when I started looking for any way I could to raise my spirits. Instantly things started improving. Money started flowing more freely, my home situation improved, and my whole demeanor transformed for the better. I started reading everything I could find that would help me understand that I am truly the creator of my own reality, and I have the choice to see things, the way I want to, through rose colored glasses.

It has been a few years now and I am still on my beautiful path. So many wonderful things have happened and I know there is so much more to come. I have learned to see things in a much more loving way and I feel good 99.9% of the time. Keeping one's self happy is a full time job and I for one am willing to make that sacrifice. I know what it feels like to be depressed and don't wish that feeling on anybody. It is very true that it all starts on the inside. And once you get the hang of happiness you can't go back. *It just feels wrong.*

My son is in his twenties now and he has a very good job, government related, and he wants so much for me to hate the government the way he does. But what he doesn't understand is that by focusing on what he hates he is just perpetuating the unwanted and making himself miserable in the meantime. He asked me, "Why won't you hate the government with me mom?" I told him it is because I want to be happy. I feel that it is easy for people to look at situations they don't agree with and try to push them away, but all that does is make it bigger and more uncomfortable for the one pushing. We can't control what other's do but we can control how we react to it. What I mean is in order to feel better about a situation you need to look at the positive side of it, or the bright side so to speak. You know there are plenty of things the government does with our tax money that is really good. They build parks and highways for us to travel on. They also provide medi-cal for people that need medical attention and can't afford it. And don't forget food stamps for families in need of assistance. There are many more things like that for us to focus on, so you get the picture. I'm sure there are things that you could think of that you appreciate about the government.

In order to see things through rose colored glasses you must see things from the bright side. Sooth your anger, fear and hate by focusing on something pleasing to you and then look for positive aspects of what you are wanting, then watch and see how much happier you are and how your world is morphing right before your very eyes, just the way you want it to.

One thing we must always remember is that we can only control our own emotions. We cannot think, act or feel for another. Nor can any other think, act or do for us. We must all find our own way to happiness, and we must find a way of staying there as often as possible. Then and only then will we truly be the beings we are meant to be. Whoa! Did that hit you like it just hit me? I hope so because I really felt a jolt. So in essence what I got from this is that by staying happy I have the power to do, be or have anything I want to. And no one or anything can project any negativity on me that I do not desire. Keeping myself focused on what I do want, and staying happy on my journey to *whatever* that is, is all my work really is. I'm going to milk this feeling for a while. It is the most clear I have been in a long time. Not that I haven't been picking up nuggets of clarity all along the way. But once in a while you get a glimpse of something that just sums up all the answers to questions that have been looming in the background, and ***BAM!, YOU KNOW!*** You just know. Right now, what I know is, that life is good and I'm doing great, and wellbeing is abundant, and it just keeps getting better as I focus and stay happy, no matter what anyone else is doing. I choose me! And I hope for all your sakes you choose **YOU!** Live the life you want no matter what anyone else thinks. They can't think for you, only you know what is right for you. And that can't be wrong. And when you live this way things will always work out for you. Remember there is great love here for you.

Your loving friend,
Deb Mertan

THAT SNEAKY DOUBT

know that it is easier said than done when someone is constantly telling you to think positive. What about all the negative things that go on every day in our lives? We grow up watching our parents worry over money or some other out of control situation, but really it's normal for things to be this way. This is where positive thinking comes in. It is our reactions to these situations that makes the difference. Think about it, what good does it do to worry or stress out about anything. In fact you are actually doing more harm than good when you react in this manner. Maybe some parents handled things with an attitude of fear and hopelessness which in turn would rub off on the children. But the ones that handled it with, "Oh, this is just another challenge to deal with", attitude, taught the children that any situation can have a silver lining. Unfortunately more parents were doom and gloom type folks so it is hard for a lot of people to see the forest for the trees.

I happened to come from a doom and gloom family. My father was a big time gambler and my mother was struck with a debilitating disease and died when I was in my early twenties. There are 5 siblings so the fighting was never ending and I couldn't wait to move out on my own to finally get some peace and quiet. When I finally did move out it gave me the calmness I needed to work on myself and find my true path in this life. I read books, learned to meditate and even joined a gym to get myself balanced in all directions. Things seemed to be going well for me in all aspects of life except in the love arena. It seemed that I was always finding guys that didn't want to fully commit to me. I felt it was because I was ahead of my time and I just needed to find someone that could understand me. I actually did get married in my early thirties, but only because I wanted children and I happened to find someone that wanted children too. I had been running my own business for about ten years at that time, and was quite successful at it so I knew that even if it didn't work out with this guy I could take care of myself and a child, so I went for it. We married and settled into a dull routine, and I stayed for twenty years. But one day I woke up and said, "I can't do this anymore". By now I was in my early fifties and I didn't want to waste any more of what was left of my youth. I still felt young and energetic and I wanted to explore life to the fullest, so I left my husband. This was at a time when the recession hit hard and I was barely making any money. I ended up in a one bathroom, three bedroom house with eight other people besides me. This was a challenge but somehow we made it work. I had two teenage children now and things got so tight that I was feeling very low and out of sorts. We were there for a year and a half before I got a call that my husband had died. It was quite a shock, but it was also a blessing in disguise. Because we were still married I got his pension and Social Security. This gave me enough money for my two kids and me to move out on our own. We were all very happy about that because it was a chance for a fresh start. We found a four bedroom house which gave me an extra room to rent out to a boarder, which in turn gave me a little more money to keep my house hold going for quite some time.

The recession was still in effect but we were doing alright for a while. Then part of the Social Security ran out and they were only giving me money for my son. I was still struggling with my business and I felt my faith fading. Not only that but my tenant moved out suddenly and that left another hole in my income. Needless to say my doom and gloom was taking over and I felt hopeless. Then my son turned eighteen and they stopped his Social Security, and that was the straw that broke the camel's back. I was sinking into a deep depression and I didn't know what I was going to do.

That wasn't the worst part, now I was being evicted from the house after two years and I didn't know if anyone else would rent to me with that on my record. I decided to do something drastic. If I was going to turn this mess around I had to feel myself with hope and faith. I began by looking up ways to lift my spirits no matter what was going on around me. I read mantras, quotes and stories of people that had been down and lifted their selves back up. I learned little tricks, like making a list of ten things I loved about myself and reading it every day before I left the house.

I would smile at myself in the mirror and say, "I love you" to my reflection. Almost instantly I found myself in a better frame of mind, it took a couple of days to really get the ball rolling, but it was rolling. At first I started noticing little things changing. Like people being extra nice to me and most of them were strangers. Then my landlord called and said he knew I was having trouble with money so he wanted to give me a month's free rent. I was astounded. Unfortunately, I was so far behind in everything that the free rent was just a minor fix, but it was the beginning of my new understanding of positive thinking. As long as I kept this up things could only get better. I made it a rule in my home that there would be no more doom and gloom and we were to all help support each other whenever one of us felt that way.

Well I fell behind in the rent again and the landlord was forced to try the eviction once again. But this time I wasn't scared and I calmly sat down to think about my options. My daughter was old enough now that she could get us a place to live in her name if it came down to it, and that's when the miracles really started to happen. All of a sudden my phone rang and it was a friend of mine that owned a rental property. She said that her tenants just gave notice that they were moving and she wanted to know if I wanted to rent her place. Well of course I said yes. By the time my court date came I was ready with a plan of action to get everything in order to go the way I wanted it to, and it did. I did not waver in my quest to get things on the right track and lo and behold everything went according to plan.

Well it has been a couple of years now since all that went down and I have to say that life just keeps getting better and better. Oh sure I have to keep reminding myself to think positive, especially when something goes awry and I start feeling that sneaky doubt try to works its way into my mind, and it will try. That is where remembering to remember that I am in control of me, not the world around me, I am in my own world, just like everyone else is in their own world. I choose to be happy and to believe that anything is possible. I have seen it with my own two eyes and I will never waver ever again no matter how events unfold in my life. In fact I have given my past life new meaning so that I can see the positive that came out of it, like if this didn't happen then that couldn't have happened. And the future is unknown so I can make it anything I want it to be. I let my life unfold a little at a time so that I don't get over anxious and worried.

It does no good to feel these ugly feelings when you could just choose to feel good all the time.

So when you choose to be happy and that sneaky doubt comes knocking on your door, just say, *"No thank you!"* and move on to the next happy thought. Just so you know I have written a whole workbook on how to get to this place in your life, it's called, **"Choose a Powerfully Positive Life"**. You can find me on the Amazon Kindle. I hope this story has given you hope that life can be exactly what you want it to be, *because it can!* So, until next time…

With all my Love, Deb Mertan

FOCUS ON THE GOOD

Have you ever noticed how the bad things in life get so much attention? Like when there is a disaster the media jumps on it and repeats it over and over again until we are inundated by it. That's all we as a whole world can think about. Like 9-11 for instance, it just about drove me into a deep depression, so much so that I literally had to stop watching and listening to all news reports. Now I'm not saying that we should ignore these awful events that come up, I'm saying that we should acknowledge that they happened and then focus on how to get things back on track in a positive way. When we keep focusing on how horrible it was we tend to bring more horrible stuff to us. Instead we should stop all repetitive news reports and talk about what we are doing to rebuild and protect our country from now on. Yes we will grieve, and rightly so. But we can't let it consume us. That's when we become weak and defenseless. I'm also not saying that we should ever forget what happened because we lost a lot of good people during that time, but we have to move on for the sake of the world. Situations like 9-11 are not the only bad things that people dwell on. What about serial killers? Why do we give them so much attention? Yes it is good to know when we need to be more cautious, but then the media takes over again and that is all that you hear about for days or even weeks sometimes. That killer is in his glory now because he is on the news and everyone knows his name. I know that is a sick way of looking at it but it's true. He wants to be recognized, and the news people give it to him. I'm not saying that it is all on the media for bringing this about because we the people are the ones buying the newspapers and watching the television broadcasts. We are giving them too much attention which in turn, in my opinion, just brings more of that behavior about. And not only do we see it on the news but then somebody thinks it's a good idea to make a movie about the crime. Oh boy, that's just more glory for the bad stuff. Do you see where I'm going with this? Look, I know that bad stuff happens all the time. Without dark there would be no light, and without bad there would be no good. We need to acknowledge it and then move on from it. If we ignore the bad we just postpone the inevitable, which is more of the bad stuff. Recognize it so that we can figure out where to go from there. We need to be aware of both sides to keep ourselves balanced.

Now let's talk about the people that focus mostly on the bad stuff. What happens is these people draw to them all the misfortune they can muster up. Not to say that these types of individuals don't have good things happen as well, but they just don't seem to realize that they are having good moments. Instead they look for what is wrong in every situation no matter how much fun they are having. They are always waiting for the other shoe to drop, so to speak. I'm here to tell you that no matter how bad things seem there is always a silver lining. You just have to analyze the situation and find it. I know that sometimes it feels impossible to feel happy, but taking deep breaths and focusing on a happy thought will bring you back to center. We need to reflect the situation so that the good will pop out at you. Have you ever been somewhere that you didn't want to be and all of a sudden you meet the one person that could help you on a project you've been working on? You look back later and realize that if you had not gone there or had left early like you had intended you would not have met this person. That's because there is something guiding you. Whether you call it God, the Universe, Buddha or any other name, it doesn't matter. If you think about it they all have the same qualities. They are invisible, they are always working for us whether we realize it or not, and we are believing without seeing. But, if you pay close attention you will see that everything you focus on, good or bad, is being given to you. So doesn't it make sense to focus more on the good things so that more of that will be given to you?

Let's take that one step further. Say you are in a situation where someone is treating you badly. How do you FEEL when this happens? If you feel pain and anger is this something you like and want? If not, do you think there is something you could do to make yourself feel good again? If all you are thinking about is how badly you are being treated then what you are doing is drawing more of that kind of situation to you. Even if you are saying that you don't want whatever it is that is bringing you sorrow you are still giving it attention. What you need to do is recognize what it is you don't want so that you can focus on what you do want. For example, if your boss is treating you badly you must stop dreading the thought of seeing them. Instead when you see their car in the parking lot say to yourself, "Oh good so-n-so is here today, I'm so happy." Pretend that you are so happy to see them that when you actually do you smile at them and act as polite as possible. Fake it 'til you make it, in other words. Have confidence in yourself. By you changing your attitude toward the situation you will change the way others perceive you. You need to go into it with a whole new mindset and in turn people will treat you better. You can use this method in any situation and it helps to have a good imagination.

As humans we can't change the way others think but we can change the way we think about ourselves. If we don't love ourselves how can we expect anyone else to truly love us? We can only take care of number one and then the rest will fall into place. If I only had one wish it would be that everyone in the world would love their self as they love their new born baby or their mother or their best friend. Not selfish love but true love. Then in turn we would all be able to love one another and life would be wonderful, just think, no more wars, instead we would have peace gatherings.

This wish is not impossible. All it will take is for each individual person to start loving their self and focusing on good things that will bring the world together as one huge family. If everyone would focus on the same wish it is totally doable. So get to it everyone. Love yourself, deeply. Allow yourself to be happy. Figure out what you want and let yourself have it. I know it sounds simple to just change the way you think, but it works. Give it a shot and see. You will be amazed and astounded at the difference it will make in your life and the lives of all people you encounter. All you have to do is change you and the rest will follow.

FYI, the Universe is always ready and willing to grant all your wishes so make them good ones. I love you all and want only the best for you. So until next time be happy and prosper.

Your Friend, Deb Mertan

BE INTENTIONAL

It's not for me to know why someone else does what they do. I can only take care of me and my journey in life. I just know that if we would all pay attention to the coincidences of our own journeys we would realize our true path and see that it's okay to switch tracks to re-invent ourselves. This is what I've come to realize about my journey, I have learned to trust my gut feelings. These deep feelings are there for a reason. It is our higher selves or the Universe or God or whoever you feel is out there helping you, trying to communicate with us. There are always signs that go along with the feelings that can show you the way to go, but you need to really pay attention. When I say be intentional, I mean to really know what it is you want in this life. Once you make it clear to your higher self, etc. you will start attracting the things and people that will help you get there. It's not always going to be the way you think it will be so you need to stay aware. For example I have always said that one day I was going to have a big house where lots of different people could come and stay and work on their own talents. But one day I realized that even though I don't have the big house YET, I always have people living with me that eventually find their true path and then move on to a happier life. It is very easy to be on the wrong path if you are not awake. You'll know when you are going astray. When you're going back to the feelings, where you don't feel secure or safe or perfect or good.

When I first started on my own new journey I was doing all the right things like my vision board, mantras, positive quotes, and thinking and talking differently. But I didn't feel like it was all happening fast enough. What I came to realize was that I wasn't feeling it deeply enough. I was feeling it but not down deep in my gut. Then one day a switch flipped in my head and I got it. I started seeing that everything that had happened up until now was happening by design, my design. I was calling everything into my life that I needed to help me learn the lessons I needed to learn to become the best me ever. It comes down to, seeing is not believing, but believing is seeing. So once we intend something, which is like asking for it, we must believe that it is ours already, and then stay alert and receive it when it comes with gratitude and joy. Another example of this in my life was when I had just gotten my washer fixed and my refrigerator was going bad, so I simply stated, as if it were already a fact, as if I had already received it, without a doubt that it was mine already, that the next thing I was going to get was a side by side refrigerator. 2 days later my roommate told me that his parents had just sold their rental house, that just happened to be very near to us, and they had a refrigerator there and we could have it if we wanted it. Of course I did. It was a white side by side and it was huge compared to my dinky frig. See, I never said the words, "buy" or "new". I just said side by side refrigerator. But seriously being specific is very helpful. I also said one night that I wished someone would come to my door with a big bag of candy and they did, but it was hard candy and I really wanted chocolate. I should have been more specific. It is the attitude and conviction that you ask for things which brings it faster and faster. And the more you see the results and believe that it is because you intended it, and for no other reason, the quicker it will manifest for you.

Now besides being intentional you must also fill yourself with love, and I mean true love which starts from within and radiates out to the Universe, to everyone and everything, and this includes our enemies. It is especially important to send love to enemies because when we hate it, just gets bigger. When we love it does the same thing, it gets bigger.

I am sure that there are some people that think there is only one way to get into heaven, but I think that there are many ways to do everything so why not heaven. When we over flow ourselves with love it has to go out and effect everyone else and then come back to us full force. Just think if everyone on earth did this, we would make living on earth as close to heaven as we could get before actually getting there. And feeling this good could only mean one thing and that is that you have to be on your right path. This is when we feel most alive and free of worry, hate, regret, negative thinking and speaking, and anything else that makes us feel bad and ugly inside.

The way I see it is that the Universe is this giant machine that runs perfectly managed by God, who has purposefully put us here on this earth to love one another. If we can do this we will be able to find the inner peace that we all seek. I know there are people that do bad things but I feel that it comes from a lack of love, and knowledge. People need to be educated about this and shown by example, as Martin Luther King Jr. showed. Even though he knew that there were people that didn't agree with him, he still kept going. The same can be said for Jesus I suppose. He was kind and loved everyone and everything even though he knew that the rulers of the day wanted to destroy everything he stood for. But he stayed true to his self and everyone else no matter what the consequences might be. The people that do the bad things are throwing a wrench into the works so to speak. But this can be stopped if all the good people start sharing their love with the Universe to spread it far and wide and to bring the harmony that we all want and need.

I feel that if we all intend for love to rule the world then it will. We need to create love circles like prayer chains. Like hands across America did only all the time not just once. That is my wish, to intentionally create a love filled Universe, so that we can all be on our right path and just be happy and filled with joy at all times. But it all starts on the inside of each and every one of us. So do yourself and everyone else a favor and look yourself in the eye in the mirror and tell yourself that you love you. It is a good place to start.

With all my love, Deb Mertan

NEW PERSPECTIVE

P eople these days are too preoccupied with the negative stuff happening all over the world right now. The news repeats everything over and over again until I want to slit my own throat, figuratively of course. I know that we need to know when bad things are happening, but I don't understand why we have to hear about it relentlessly, until people start feeling scared to walk out of their own homes. And we can't blame the media for putting it out there because by us watching it on CNN or whatever news channel you prefer, we are saying, "So give us more bad news, that's what we want to hear about."

Now, if you believe in the Law of Attraction, and I do, you have to see that by focusing on this bad stuff we are just getting more bad stuff. I know many of you may be thinking, "What can I do, I am only one person." But if every "one person" stopped watching the news and reading newspapers it would send a big fat message to the media to change things up. There are plenty of good things happening in our world too. We need to give a majority of our attention to the good stuff and only glimpse at the bad stuff for comparison or reference. There should be only two times per day that you get updated on the bad news. Once in the morning and once in the early evening. That way you have time to shake it off before you go to sleep at night. Whatever we hear last is probably what our subconscious mind will dwell on while we sleep. And having the bad news only twice a day can give the media a chance to research what they are talking about and give true facts. Have you ever really listened to some of these reporters when they say things like, "I think he may have meant this", and then they give their false opinion on the

subject. That sticks in people's minds and then the rumors start to get around and everything goes haywire. We need real facts so that we can all make educated decisions on what we want to believe.

Another thing that the media could do is have a love moment every hour or so. What I mean by this is, they have so much power and access to the world that if they started a love moment and had everyone watching; close their eyes and send loving energy to the whole world, especially to our enemies, the vibe of the whole Universe would change and we would see people getting along and truly loving one another.

The Law of Attraction says that what we focus on the most is what will come to us. Whether it's good or bad we will bring it to ourselves, so why not make it good. Love attracts love, while hate and fear only attracts more hate and fear. How simple is that?

Science and religion are now starting to come together. God would not have let us know science if it wasn't going to be useful. This is bringing a sense of new found spirituality to the world. People are seeing that by changing the way they think and speak it is causing a change in consciousness. Science has proven through quantum physics that our minds are very powerful and if we learn to use them more efficiently we will all live much happier and more fulfilling lives. Our part of this is to research everything ourselves and not just automatically believe everything we hear. People lie and distort the truth, but these days we have more information than ever right at our fingertips, through internet, books, You Tube videos, and numerous other places. There is no reason these days for rumors to get out of hand. Start watching videos on quantum physics and metaphysical quantum physics and you will be amazed at what you find. We are all energy and we are all connected. We can change the spirituality of the world if we all focus on the good. You have to say what you mean and mean what you say. Be honest and forthright. Send fear packing and send love to everyone and everything every day. Get to know who you really are, and if you are not who you want to be then become the person you want to be. Individually we all need to do our part so that we can come together as one world. I have been becoming myself for quite some time now and I just love myself more and more as I learn about what I really want. My life has changed so drastically for the better that I just have to share it with all who are reading this blog. I would love nothing more than to see the world come together as one and end hunger and suffering and all wars once and for all. I hope that this message spreads like wild fire and we all start focusing on the good. Have a new perspective.

Love, Deb

MAKE A DECISION ALREADY!

Clarity is so liberating. Life is like a smorgasbord of things to choose from and when we feel unsure or out of sorts in some way it can feel very uncomfortable. As you may have noticed I have used the word "feel" a couple of times already and will be using it a lot more throughout this blog. When we are in between decisions we should give ourselves a little time to focus on each direction, even if there are several choices. We will know by the way we feel what is right for us at that moment. In reality there is no wrong direction. No matter which way we go it will all lead to the place we really want to be. One way just may take a little longer than another way. We must also realize that there is never just one way to do anything. And you may get to see and experience things you wouldn't have if you took the other direction. But getting back to feeling, once you make a solid decision you feel better and ideas can flow more easily and you will be undergoing a very good journey. In actuality you are always on your right path but at times you may be going slower and other times you may be moving with the speed of light. Then again when we find ourselves dwelling on our miseries we may feel like we are swimming or paddling our boat upstream. It will seem very hard and not very enjoyable.

I want to tell you a little story about something that at that moment seemed like a disaster but turned out to be a pretty good day. One day I was driving down the freeway with my 7 year old daughter and my 3 year old son. As I was coming to the end of the off ramp there was a loud explosion. I had no idea what it could be. Suddenly black smoke was bellowing out from underneath my van so naturally I thought it was on fire. I jumped out and yelled at the kids to get out but they kept arguing about who should go first. I just reached in and pulled them out myself. Before I knew it there were about 4 firemen there with extinguishers that came from the fire station from across the street. It turned out that my transmission just blew a hole out the top and all the fluid came out causing the black smoke. I actually got back in the van and drove it to a gas station down the street where my brother-in-law was waiting for us. As soon as we pulled into the parking lot the van died completely. Of course we had to call a tow truck to come and take all of us to my favorite mechanic shop. From there we called a taxi cab to come and take us home. While in my mind I was thinking that this was a terrible day my little 3 year old son looked up at me and said, "We're on an adventure, huh mom". Suddenly things didn't seem so bad and I said, "Yes we are son". Because he showed me a whole new perspective and made me laugh, things instantly got better.

Our mindset needs to be adjusted just like the knob on the radio dial. We need to tune to the station that feels good to us. And sometimes we may feel that we are out of sync or even starting from scratch, but that is just the Universe saying, "Wake up you're swimming upstream". Once we switch back to the station that feels good then life will once again start to unfold in ways we never even imagined it could. Sometimes you will hear the most profound statements in movies too, like "The Santa Clause" with Tim Allen. I love the scene where he is at the North Pole talking to Judy the elf, saying, "I see it but I don't believe it". She says that most adults forget because they grow out of the belief, but that kids just know, because seeing is not believing, believing is seeing. Or the movie "Halloween Town" with Debbie Reynolds. She is flying on her broom stick with her grand-daughter on the back and the grand-daughter asks her how magic works. She says something to the effect of, I just think of what I want and then I let myself have it. Whatever we focus on the most is what is going to manifest in our lives whether it is good or bad. So don't you think it is better to focus on what you do want rather than the lack of it? There are always signs and most of it comes through our feelings. I know that it can seem a little weird or uncomfortable to change the way you have been feeling. But if you really think about it everything that is new to you was uncomfortable at first. When you first learned to ride a bike or drive a car or especially use a computer, it was weird and uncomfortable, right? But now it is so easy you don't even have to think about it. That is exactly what happens when we start being more deliberate and more decisive. At first we have to consciously recognized that we are in that wobbly undecided mode, then we can deliberately make a decision and try it out for a couple of days and see how it feels. The beauty in this is that if it doesn't feel good we can always change the station and go in another direction. See, it's a failsafe design.

Another thing that doesn't feel good is when we are being judged, especially by ourselves, or judging others. That kind of thinking only holds us back or causes us to be going upstream again, which only delays the good stuff. When I find myself thinking in this manner I have to ask the question, "What would unconditional love do?" There is no judgment in unconditional, so if we just love we will see that that is the only way to truly bring joy into our own hearts. That joy will radiate out into the Universe and cause an avalanche of happiness to all that come in contact with you. Then you will be flowing down stream again until the next time something feels off.

Even though words can't really teach, they can evoke feelings that help bring all your desires to fruition. And once you get a taste of the happiness and joy that comes with being true to yourself and making the decisions that turn you on and excite you to go forward, you can never go back. Sometimes life doesn't turn out like you thought it would, sometimes it turns out better. So enjoy the roller coaster ride and go with the flow, whatever that may be for you.

With all my Love,
Deb Mertan

ABOUT THE AUTHOR

My name is Deb Mertan and I am a very happy person. But I haven't always been this person. I was in a bad marriage and it was an unhappy time in my life. I actually left my husband and started divorce procedures, but before that could happen I became a widow. And to make matters worse this was the beginning of the recession in 2008. After that was all over it seemed like I couldn't find happiness or at least not for very long. Things just kept getting worse. My kids were having trouble in school and I couldn't handle it. I was depressed and cried a lot. I couldn't keep up on the rent or even buy school clothes for my kids. I was a mess. It wasn't until I saw the fear in my children's eyes that I finally snapped out of my depression. I decided I wasn't being my true self and I had to find a way to lift my spirits. I knew I could be a much better person so I went on the internet and looked up processes to help me change my mind set about myself. One of the first exercises I did was I wrote a list of ten things I loved about myself. This is something I learned was not as easy as it sounds. So I wrote things like, "I love that freckle on my toe, or I love that I love my kids". This may not seem very important but it got the ball rolling because I was using the word love toward myself. I would re-write the list every seven days and I would only read it to myself once a day in the morning before I started my day. This started working and I saw things changing very quickly.

Then I learned about, "The Secret". I studied what they were saying on the CD's for quite a while and things got a little better but it wasn't working the way I thought it should. Then one day I was visiting a friend and she mentioned Abraham Hicks. I asked who that was and she gasped. Right away she pulled up a pod cast and as I listened I knew this was the missing piece. From that time on I have been listening to these pod casts every day.

This is when I truly understood the Law of Attraction. This is when things really started changing. I bought a new car and I actually bought a house. I started a web page too, www.loveequalslove.org, and I write inspirational blogs of true stories of what my friends and I have been doing to make our dreams come true, because the Law of Attraction is working for all of us all the time.

I know now that by keeping myself in a good mood makes all the difference in the world. And now that I know this I can never go back to that sad miserable person. I know too much now. That is why I decided to put some of my blogs in a book to help anyone who wants to feel better and get an idea of how this all works. I want to share stories of myself and people I know personally and let you see for yourself how it can work for you too.

I hope you enjoy these uplifting tales and find your happiness as well.

With Great Love,
Deb Mertan